Career Guide to the Animal Health Field

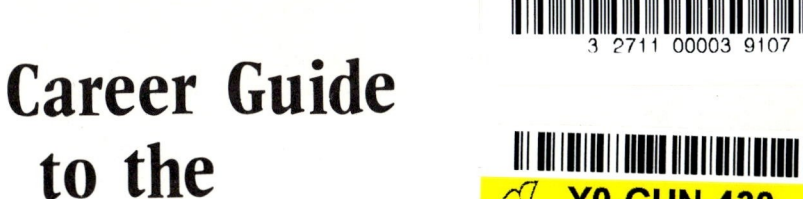

by
M. Leigh Simmons, DVM

HARWAL
publishing co.
326 west state st.
media, pa. 19063

ACKNOWLEDGEMENT

I would like to acknowledge the invaluable assistance of Ann M. Campbell, Director of Training, Program Resources, Inc, The National Center for Toxicological Research, Jefferson, Arkansas in the preparation of Chapters Five, Six and Seven.

M.L.S.

Copyright © 1980 by Harwal Publishing Company
Library of Congress Catalog Card No. 79-90139
ISBN 0-932036-01-5
All rights reserved
First Edition
Manufactured in the United States of America

Photo credits
Oklahoma State University

Preface

It seems that everyone I talk to has a son, daughter, niece, nephew, or neighbor who wants to be a veterinarian. I am often asked by people how they should go about getting into a veterinary school; what is necessary in terms of scholastic preparation. And a thousand other questions!

It is not my purpose to persuade anyone to, or to dissuade anyone from, being a veterinarian. This book is presented simply to provide information about the subject so that it will be easier for the individual to reach a career decision.

Information concerning specific veterinary schools, and pre-veterinary medicine curriculums are included here. Also discussed is what the veterinary field offers in a wide range of career options within the profession.

Importantly, alternatives to the career of the doctor of veterinary medicine are presented. The allied fields of the animal technologist and the animal technician are examined in depth.

There is currently a crisis in veterinary education. The expanding role of veterinary medicine in mitigating society's major health threats, and the emerging role of the profession in ecology, space biology, and world food production, emphasize an already critical shortage of veterinarians. There are now about 30,000 active veterinarians in the United States. Based on recommendations of the Senate Committee on Government Operations, 40,075 veterinarians will be required to satisfy public need in the United States in the 1980's. The validity of this estimate has recently been confirmed through an extensive study by a committee of the National Academy of Sciences. Unless enrollment in colleges of veterinary medicine increases substantially, only 32,000 veterinarians will be available in the country in the early 1980's, a projected shortage of about 8,000. The addition of three veterinary schools has eased the problem, but a total of three or four additional colleges will be needed to meet the demand by the year 2000.

All existing colleges of veterinary medicine have recently expanded their teaching programs, and several states and groups of states are developing a new veterinary school. In time, the new and expanded facilities probably will be able to educate enough veterinarians to overcome the shortage. For students who are able to get into a college of veterinary medicine and complete the program, the employment outlook is good.

Money magazine states, "Doctors, dentists, and veterinarians enjoy the unique advantages of a strong assured growth combined with a limited supply of new blood." The Bureau of Labor Statistics estimates that the United States needs about 22,000 new physicians a year, but the American medical schools are turning out only about 15,000. The number of medical schools has increased from 103 in 1970 to 120 today. Six more schools are being established, so the supply of new doctors is coming closer to the demand. After 1985, there might even be a surplus. Nevertheless, during the next several years there will still be a gap. Moreover, the Health Professions Educational Assistance Act of 1976 has reduced the immigration of foreign-trained doctors who helped bridge that gap.

The growth in demand for dentists and veterinarians will be somewhat less than that for physicians. However, these professions will also experience a shortage.

The need for other kinds of medical workers is growing just as fast as the professions, but since the supply of qualified people is ample, the compensation remains relatively poor.

Money magazine lists veterinarians under "Professions with a Promise" and estimates a 27% growth in jobs by the mid 1980's. Therefore, prospects for qualified job seekers are excellent.

Table of Contents

Chapter 1
WHAT
DO VETERINARIANS ACTUALLY DO?...................... 1

Chapter 2
PREPARATION
FOR VETERINARY SCHOOL............................. 9

Chapter 3
DOCTORAL PROGRAM
OF VETERINARY MEDICINE............................13

Chapter 4
COLLEGES OF
VETERINARY MEDICINE
ADMISSION POLICIES...............................19

Chapter 5
INTRODUCTION TO
ALLIED ANIMAL HEALTH CAREERS.....................97

Chapter 6
ANIMAL HEALTH
TECHNOLOGY PROGRAMS.............................107

Chapter 7
LABORATORY HEALTH TECHNICIAN....................117

CHAPTER 1
What Do Veterinarians Actually Do?

Many people see the veterinarian in only one role, that of the veterinary practitioner. There are, however, many other opportunities open.

Today, well over 30,000 veterinarians are professionally active in the United States. They provide a wide variety of services in private practice, teaching and research, regulatory medicine, public health, military service, private industry, and other specialized activities.

The American Veterinary Medical Association recognizes the following professional specialties: State Licensed Practices:
- Mixed practice (50%-50% large and small animals)
- Mixed practice (over 50% large animals)
- Mixed practice (over 50% small animals)
- Small animal practice (exclusive)
- Large animal practice (all species)
- Equine practice (exclusive)
- Bovine practice (exclusive)
- Porcine practice (exclusive)
- Poultry practice (exclusive)

PRIVATE PRACTICE

In private practice, veterinarians strive to prevent disease and other health problems. They examine their animal patients, immunize them against diseases, and advise owners on ways to keep pets and livestock healthy.

When problems do occur, the practitioner must diagnose and treat the patient. Accurate diagnosis frequently requires the use of laboratory tests, X-rays, and specialized equipment. Treatment may involve a number of procedures such as administering emergency lifesaving measures, prescribing medication, setting a fracture, performing surgery, or counseling the owner on care and feeding.

Records of the American Veterinary Medical Association show that about seventy-six percent of the veterinarians in the United States are in private practice. About thirty-five percent of the veterinarians in this country engage in small animal practice; they treat only pet animals, mostly dogs and cats.

Approximately seven percent are exclusively in large animal practice, specializing in the care of farm animals and horses.

Another thirty-four percent are involved in what is known a mixed animal practice. Their patients may include all types of pets, horses and livestock.

Veterinarians in private practice are responsible for the health of approximately 150 million cattle, some 155 million hogs, and about 15 million sheep, which help make up the nation's $40,000,000,000 livestock industry. Also, they care for more than 8 million horses, as well as cat and dog populations estimated to number at least 30 million each.

MILITARY VETERINARY MEDICINE

United States Army and Air Force veterinarians comprise a small proportion of the total national resource of veterinarians. The Services have an annual requirement of about sixty-five veterinarians. Almost one-third of the veterinary medical profession is employed in areas other than clinical practice, notably in public health, regulatory medicine, and biomedical research. This is readily apparent in the utilization of veterinarians in the military medical departments where veterinary officers are involved more with military community health protection than with animal health care.

Military food safety and quality are among the

essential responsibilities of the military veterinarian, although many of the actual services are provided by highly trained enlisted technicians under officer supervision. Because of transportation and lengthy storage requirements, stringent demands are placed upon the quality and longevity of foods for the military - much more stringent, in fact, than those placed upon civilian food. In oversea areas, and especially in wartime, the military veterinary service is responsible for the entire inspection process, including the health of livestock prior to slaughter, through final issuance of the food product to troop units. The control of diseases naturally transmitted between animals and man, and the prevention of foodborne disease are vital elements in the military community health program. The veterinarian's training in basic medical sciences, with emphasis on public health, epidemiology, parasitology and food hygiene, qualifies him for expanded responsibilities in these areas of preventive medicine.

Military regulations also require certain animal disease prevention and control measures for privately owned animals of service members as a part of the preventive medicine and military community health programs.

Beyond the regulatory work, military veterinarians engage in biomedical and subsistence research and development. They have contributed to our understanding of many important diseases, and to the development and improvements of surgical prostheses and innovations. Veterinary officers with specialized training in laboratory animal medicine maintain animal colonies to assure that properly conditioned and disease-free animals are available and utilized in accordance with regulatory standards and ethical practices. Other government-owned animals such as sentry, scout, tracker, and drug-detection dogs, and a small number of horses and mules receive complete veterinary medical and surgical care.

Military veterinarians provide indispensable professional services to other governmental agencies both within and outside the Department of Defense. The Navy and Marine Corps are provided services by the veterinary staffs of the Army and Air Force. The United States Department of Agriculture has received timely and vital support from the Services, and particularly from the veterinary officers of the Army and Air Force, as in the National Animal Disease Emergencies of 1971 (VEE) and 1972 (Exotic Newcastle Disease). Many military veterinary officers are certified as Diplomates in one of the specialties recognized by the American Veterinary Medical Association. These specialties include veterinary pathology, public health, microbiology, surgery and laboratory animal medicine.

REGULATORY VETERINARY MEDICINE

Regulatory veterinary medicine is the medical practice that is under the control of law or constituted authority which treats the diseases and injuries of animals.

VETERINARY PUBLIC HEALTH

Veterinary public health is the science dealing with the protection and improvement of animal health.

TEACHING AND RESEARCH

In teaching and research, veterinarians strive to expand their profession's knowledge of health and disease, and to assure that its members have the best possible preparation for providing the many services society requires of them.

Nearly 2,000 veterinarians are needed to educate tomorrow's veterinarians at the twenty-four American colleges of veterinary medicine accredited by the

American Veterinary Medical Association. In addition to teaching, veterinary school faculty members conduct research, contribute to scientific publications and develop continuing education programs to help practitioners acquire new knowledge and techniques.
    Research veterinarians working for private firms, colleges and government agencies are seeking better ways to prevent and solve animal health problems. Many animal and human ailments such as cancer and cardiovascular disease are studied with the help of experimental animals which are carefully bred, raised, and maintained under the supervision of veterinarians. Laboratory animal veterinarians help select the best animal models for particular experiments, and assure that they are properly cared for.
    In addition to developing ways to reduce or eliminate the threat of many animal diseases, veterinarians involved in research have made many direct contributions to human health. These include discoveries which helped conquer malaria and yellow fever, solved the mystery of botulism (a type of food poisoning), and produced an anti-coagulent used to treat some types of heart disease.

MISCELLANEOUS SPECIALTIES

    In addition to the major specialty divisions of veterinary medicine, there are numerous other areas of study in which a veterinarian can ve involved. They are:
    Fur bearing animals
    Zoo animals (animals collected for display)
    Laboratory animal medicine - the science of
       treating disease in experimental animals
    Diagnostic Veterinary Medicine - the medical
       practice which determines the nature of the
       disease of animals.
    Within veterinary schools, government, the food and drug industry, as well as many other industries,

there are veterinarians who devote their time particularly to one of the following fields:
- Anatomy – the branch of morphology which studies the structure of animals or plants, and the relation of their parts
- Biochemistry – the chemistry of living tissues
- Microbiology – the biology of microorganisms
- Nutrition – the sum of the processes concerned in the growth, maintenance, and repair of the living body as a whole, or of its constituent parts
- Ophthalmology – the science and study of the anatomy, physiology and diseases of the eye
- Parasitology – the science and study of organisms that obtain nourishment at the expense of the host on, or in, which they live
- Pathology (Avian) – the branch of biological science which deals with the nature of the diseases of birds
- Pathology (clinical) – the diagnosis of disease by laboratory methods
- Pathology (general) – a study of disturbances that are common to various tissues and organs of the body
- Pharmacology – the science of the nature and properties of drugs, particularly the actions of drugs
- Physiology – the science that deals with the functions of living organisms or their parts
- Radiology – the branch of medicine that deals with radioactive substances, X-rays, and other ionizing radiations, and with their utilization in the diagnosis and treatment of disease
- Surgery – the branch of medicine dealing with trauma and diseases requiring operative procedure, including manipulation
- Toxicology – the science of the nature and effects of poisons, their detection, and treatment of their effects.

In addition, there are specialties, or combinations of specialties, that are not listed in the AVMA classifications:
- Research - studious inquiry or examination of tissues, systems molecules, or biochemical reactions
- Veterinary Medical Writing and Editing - in all types of veterinary publications, such as textbooks and periodicals
- Industrial Management - particularly in pharmaceutical companies
- Marine Biology - the study of sea life, its functions, its diseases, and its uses
- Biomedical Engineering - the engineering of buildings, systems, and equipment to be used in biomedical research or in clinical medicine
- Animal Facility Designing
- Animal Caging and Equipment Designing.

Within the last several years, the following specialties have been added to the AVMA classifications:
- Theriogenlology - an account of the descent of an animal group from an ancestor of older forms
- Veterinary Internal Medicine - the nonsurgical management of diseases in animals
- Anesthesiology - the art and science of administering local and general anesthetics to produce the various types of anesthesia.

CHAPTER 2
Preparation for Veterinary School

HIGH SCHOOL

A surprising number of students make up their mind as to their ultimate profession while they are still in high school, some even earlier. In general, a young person who hopes to become a veterinarian should be an excellent student, with an inquiring mind and keen powers of observation. Aptitude for, and a deep interest in, biological sciences are essential. A veterinarian must like and understand animals. Equally important is the ability to understand and get along well with people. Compassion for people as well as for animals is perhaps the most valuable asset a veterinarian can possess.

There are numerous ways that high school students can begin to build experience which will be of value to them - not only in seeking acceptance into veterinary school, but during their veterinary schooling as well.

Farm backgrounds are, of course, ideal. But today fewer and fewer veterinarians come from a rural background. Any association with animals is beneficial. Possibilities are dog breeding, dog training, cat breeding, cat showing, rabbit breeding, and hamster breeding. At least one of these is practical for almost everyone.

One might also consider part-time work in pet shops, dairies, stables, race-tracks, meat packing plants, with chicken growers and the like. It is a rare individual who does not live near a venture that involves animals or animal by-products. It is equally true that most of the people in these industries will welcome reliable, interested part-time help.

Often it is possible to arrange summertime vacation and weekend work. Also, some areas have excellent 4-H programs (involving animals) which are of value.

In terms of academic work in high school, it is best to keep all options open. In general, any medical profession - veterinary medicine, dentistry, human medicine - requires the same pre-med preparation at the college level. Therefore, it is best in high school to take as much biology, chemistry, physics, and mathematics as possible. Modern day medicine of all kinds involves very sophisticated electronic equipment and utilizes numerous computerized programs; it is useful to take related courses, if available.

Obviously, high school is none too soon to begin to build a broad base of knowledge for the future. If later, the individual decides to go into another field, medical or otherwise, he or she will still be in an excellent position.

COLLEGE

In order to become a veterinarian, a person must complete at least six years of college education, and earn a Doctor of Veterinary Medicine (DVM) degree or its equivalent. A four-year professional course of study leading to this degree is offered by twenty-five colleges in the United States. Each school is evaluated regularly by the American Veterinary Medical Association, and must maintain high standards of excellence in order to keep its accreditation.

To be considered for admission to a college of veterinary medicine, a student must first complete a minimum of two years, and for some colleges, three years of pre-veterinary medical study. Each college of veterinary medicine prescribes its own pre-veterinary requirements. Typically, these include basic language arts, social sciences, humanities, and course work in mathematics, biological and physical sciences.

Pre-veterinary coursework can be taken at many

universities, including those at which the veterinary medical schools are located. However, a student should check with the professional school to which he or she plans to apply, and make certain that credit will be given for pre-veterinary courses that have been taken elsewhere.

It is advantageous to take pre-med training at the same campus where the veterinary college is located. This, of course, is not always possible, but would allow one to have access to much more information about that particular school.

Although an individual must work within the specific requirements of the university attended, it is wise to fill all elective courses with substantial technological study. The more that is known when a person enters veterinary school, the more he or she will enjoy the years spent there. It is a poor time to have to "catch-up" or "fill gaps."

CHAPTER 3
Doctoral Program of Veterinary Medicine

VETERINARY SCHOOL

In most colleges of veterinary medicine, the professional program is divided into two phases. During the first phase (generally, the first two years), pre-clinical sciences, including anatomy, physiology, pathology, pharmacology, and microbiology are emphasized. Most of the student's time is spent in classroom and laboratory study.

The second phase (the third and fourth years) of professional study is largely clinical. During much of this time students work with animal patients and deal with owners who use the school's clinical services. The clinical curriculum includes courses on infectious and non-infectious diseases, advanced pathology, applied anatomy, obstetrics, radiology, clinical medicine, and surgery. Students also study public health, preventive medicine, toxicology, nutrition, professional ethics, and business practices.

For most people, veterinary medical study is difficult. Students must learn and remember hundreds of terms and facts about many different animals and diseases. They must also become skilled in surgical techniques, and many laboratory and diagnostic procedures.

A typical veterinary student spends approximately 5,000 hours in classroom, laboratory, and clinical study. And, because the time required for instruction takes up practically all of a student's day, many more hours must be spent at night and on weekends doing lengthy reading assignments, additional laboratory research, library research, and independent study. Leisure time is a scare commodity.

BEYOND VETERINARY SCHOOL

In many ways, a veterinarian's education only begins with a DVM degree. New scientific knowledge and techniques are constantly being developed, and a veterinarian must keep up to date by reading scientific journals and attending professional meetings, short courses, and seminars.

Before a veterinarian can engage in private practice in any state, he or she must also have a license issued by that state. A license is granted only to veterinarians who pass rigid state board examinations to prove they are competent to serve the public. Veterinarians in most states are not required to complete an internship before going into practice. Even so, many intership and residency programs do exist, and increasing numbers of veterinarians are taking advantage of them. For example, there is an active internship program in the State of Oregon by which a new graduate, wishing to practice in that state, must work for one year with a licensed practitioner before he or she is eligible to practice on their own. Other possibilities exist for advanced study by working in a veterinary school, humane shelter, and the like while taking advanced study in the specialty of one's choice.

A number of non-practice positions in government agencies and commercial firms do not require a license, although many veterinarians who take these jobs do have one.

HOW TO GET INTO A COLLEGE OF VETERINARY MEDICINE

Is it hard to get into veterinary school?
Yes.
Veterinary medical education requires expensive clinical and laboratory facilities, many live animal patients, and a great deal of individual instruction.

The cost of educating a veterinarian is high, and most of the funds used for this purpose must come from state and federal government sources. As a result, just twenty-five universities in this country have established a college of veterinary medicine.

Completion of a pre-veterinary program does not guarantee admission to a college of veterinary medicine. For the past several years, many more students have applied than the professional schools have had room for. Nationwide, United States colleges of veterinary medicine are now able to accept only about fifteen percent of all qualified applicants.

As has been discussed, anyone who hopes to get into a college of veterinary medicine must complete a prescribed course of pre-veterinary study with high grades. Practical experience or extra years of college is very helpful. But, because educational facilities are limited, many capable people who want to enter the profession never have a chance to study veterinary medicine.

Since it is so difficult to get into a college of veterinary medicine, a student who plans to apply should select an alternate career in case his or her application is turned down. In fact, many veterinary schools suggest this in their literature concerning admissions. With careful planning, the courses needed to meet pre-veterinary requirements should also provide suitable preparation for a number of alternate careers.

Usually, if you are a resident of a state that has its own veterinary school, you are more likely to be accepted into that school than one in another state. If you live in a state that does not have its own school, there is a possibility that your state has a quota agreement established with a veterinary school in another state. Naturally, though, you will be competing for a smaller number of openings. If it is possible, you should establish residence in the state of the veterinary college of your choice, and it should be done well in advance of your applying to the school.

Specific admissions requirements, school by school, are detailed in the following chapter. All Amercian colleges of veterinary medicine are included, and all are AVMA approved.

EDUCATIONAL COMMISSION FOR FOREIGN VETERINARY GRADUATES CERTIFICATION PROGRAM

Graduation from an accredited or approved college of veterinary medicine is a requirement of most state licensing agencies for eligibility to sit for licensing examinations. It is also a requirement for employment as a veterinarian by most government agencies. At present, only veterinary colleges in the United States and Canada are accredited. Many state licensing agencies and other government agencies accept, in lieu of graduation from an accredited college, the ECFVG (Educational Commission for Foreign Veterinary Graduates) Certificate, as issued by the AVMA.

ECFVG certificates are issued upon satisfactory completion of the four steps listed below.
1) Proof of graduation from a college of veterinary medicine
2) Proof of comprehension and ability to communicate in the English language. Applicants who have graduated from a United States or Canadian secondary school where the language of instruction is English will not be required to take the English examination.
3) Proof of having attained a passing score on the ECFVG examination in veterinary medicine
4) Proof of successful completion of a year of evaluated clinical experience at a site approved by ECFVG.

Further details can be obtained by writing to:

ECFVG
American Veterinary Medical Association
930 North Meacham Road
Schaumburg, Illinois 60172

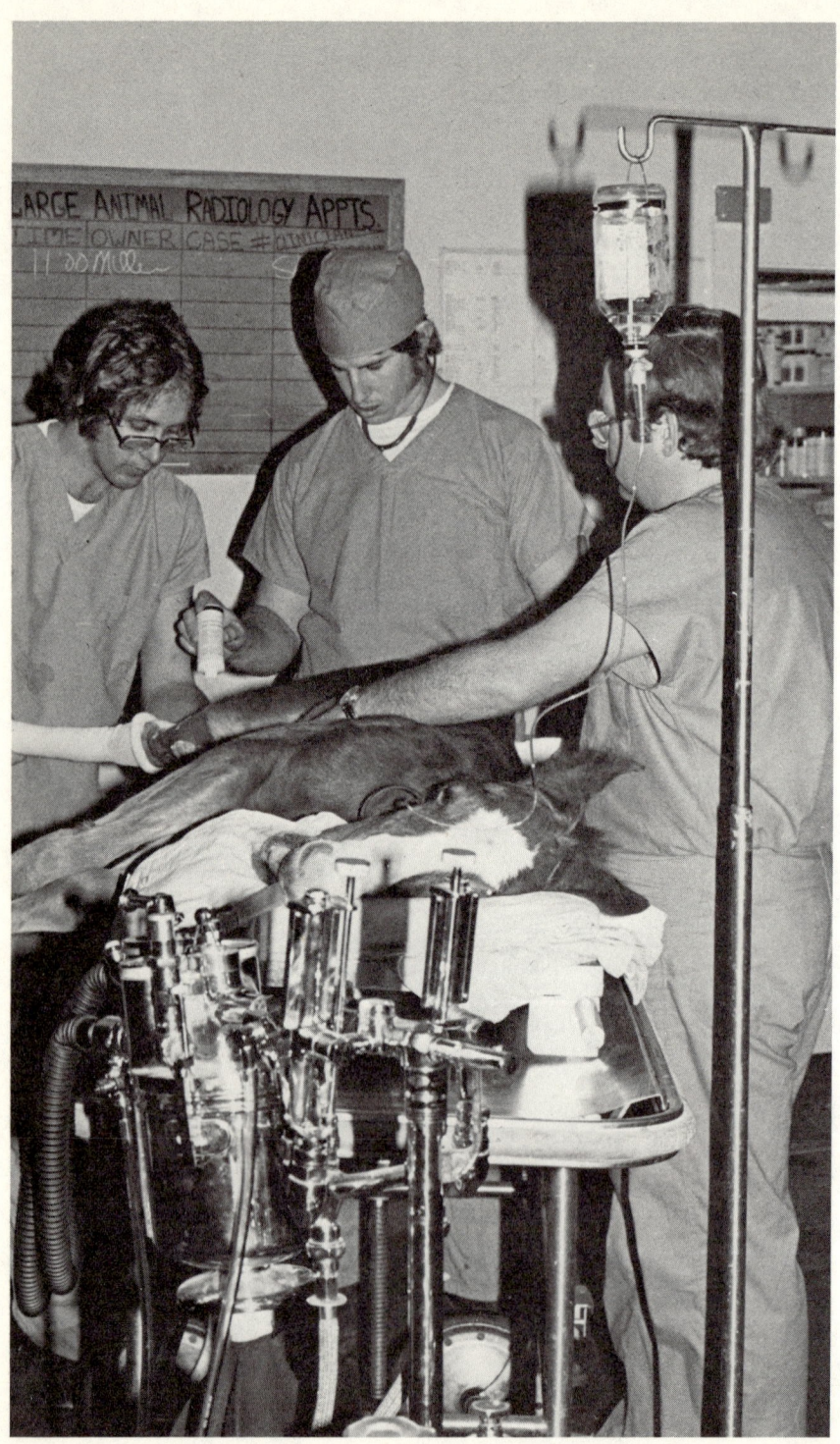

CHAPTER 4
Colleges of Veterinary Medicine Admission Policies

AUBURN UNIVERSITY
School of Veterinary Medicine
Auburn, Alabama 36830

The Auburn University founded the College of Veterinary Medicine in 1907 from a division of veterinary science and physiology, which was established in 1892. The name was changed to School of Veterinary Medicine in 1927.

From 1907 to 1916, the professional curriculum covered three years of nine months each; in 1917 it was increased to four years.

At first, entrance was by certificate from an accredited high school or by examination in high school subjects. In 1912, the entrance requirements were increased to 12 units or three years of high school; in 1914 to 14 units; and in 1921 to 15 units or the successful completion of an examination of four years of high school work. In 1935, graduation from an accredited high school plus one year, or a minimum of 30 semester hours of college work, was required. Effective with the academic year 1968-69, seven quarters of study in an accredited college or university were required. These seven quarters must represent 123 quarter hours or 82 semester hours. The minimum acceptable grade point average is 1.25, based on the A=3 scale.

Admission Requirements

The southern states, through contracts with the Southern Regional Education Board are cooperating in providing graduate and professional education. Auburn

University's School of Veterinary Medicine serves four states: Alabama, Kentucky, North Carolina and Virginia. While there is no limit on applications, the School's facilities make it necessary to restrict admissions.

The land-grant institutions in each state participating under the Southern Regional Education plan maintains a counseling and guidance service for students who desire admission the the School of Veterinary Medicine. Students attending other than land-grant institutions of the participating states should contact the counseling and guidance service in their state for information and advice concerning the specific courses which will be acceptable in the pre-veterinary curriculum. Inquiries should be made early in the student's educational career. Address inquiries to:

Alabama:
    Dean, School of Arts and Sciences, or
    Dean, School of Agriculture
    Auburn University
    Auburn, Alabama 36830

Kentucky:
    Executive Secretary
    Council on Public Higher Education
    Capital Plaza Office Tower
    Frankfort, Kentucky 40601

North Carolina:
    Director of Academic Affairs
    Agricultural and Life Sciences
    111 Patterson Hall
    North Carolina State University
    Raleigh, North Carolina 27605

Virginia
   Coordinator
   Commonwealth of Virginia
   Council of Higher Education
   700 Fidelity Building
   9th and Main Sts.
   Richmond, Virginia 23219

The procedure for residency certification varies among states served by the SREB, but residency must have been established at the time of application. In considering Alabama applicants, the length of residence will also be a factor.

The minimum academic requirement for admission to the School of Veterinary Medicine is the satisfactory completion of all courses listed in the first seven quarters of the pre-veterinary program of the Auburn Bulletin. Courses taken at other institutions must be the exact equivalent of these courses. A total of 123 quarter hours or 82 semester hours of college credit must be completed with an honor point average of at least 1.50 based on an A=3 honor points. A grade of "D" on required courses will not be accepted. In addition, applicants are required to meet the physical training requirements in effect at the institution attended. Transfer students who have not met the physical education requirements of the institution from which they transfer will be required to arrange to clear any shortages at Auburn University at the time of admission.

The Committee sets no age limit on entering students, but priority decreases in relation to the diminishing number of productive years following graduation. The preferred age for applicants is 20 to 28 years. Only in exceptional circumstances will applicants older than 30 years be considered for admission. Currently, the average entering student's age is 23.

UNIVERSITY OF CALIFORNIA
School of Veterinary Medicine
Davis, California 95616

The University of California organized a college of veterinary medicine in 1894 at the affiliated colleges on the San Francisco campus. Several classes and a total of eighteen students were graduated. Because of meager enrollment, the college was closed in 1900. A department of veterinary science was established in the College of Agriculture on the University of California Berkeley campus in 1901 where the personnel devoted time to research in the agricultural experiment station.

The present School of Veterinary Medicine, situated on the Davis campus, opened in the fall of 1948 with forty-two students. From 1949 through 1964 classes of fifty-two students were admitted. Commencing in 1965 the entering class was eighty students, but was increased to eighty-five in 1970 and to ninety-four in 1972. The first class was graduated in June, 1952.

Admission Requirements

In view of the pressures from residents of the State of California for admission to the School of Veterinary Medicine, it is the stated policy of the Unversity that, with only rare exceptions, admission to the School is limited to residents of the State. There are five to six applications from residents for admission to each of the ninety-four first-year places in the DVM curriculum each year, and it is virtually impossible for a California resident to gain admission to a veterinary school elsewhere.

In cases where admissions exceptions are made, first preference is given to residents of states participating in the Western Interstate Commission for Higher Education (WICHE). For this reason, an application form will be available only to residents and students from WICHE states.

The first academic step for admission to be completed consists of a series of required courses which can be taken in any accredited college or university where they are offered. Most credits for courses taken in accredited community or state colleges and/or universities can be accepted by the University of California. The applicant should determine from the Associate Dean of Student Services of the School of Veterinary Medicine which credits will be accepted by the University of California, Davis. One must be careful to select courses comparable or similar to those described in the catalog.

Applicants must have completed the equivalent of at least three full academic years in an accredited college or university, and fulfilled 135 quarter course units (90 semester course units) before entering the School of Veterinary Medicine.

All applicants are required to take the Aptitude Test and Advanced Test in Biology of the Graduate Record Examination (GRE).

Demonstration of outstanding academic achievement is a necessary prerequisite for admission to the professional veterinary medical curriculum. Applicants are advised that the grade point averages of classes admitted in the last five years have ranged from 3.2 to 3.6.

Non-academic requirements for admission consist of the applicant's narrative, stated animal experience, and letters of evaluation. The non-academic record will be evaluated for the applicant's understanding of the profession and the responsibilities of being a veterinarian, interest in serving the public through the profession of veterinary medicine, maturity, motivation, and those other qualities necessary for successful academic and professional work. Substantial experience with animals, which may include working with veterinarians, is required. That experience should entail more than having had familty pets. Letters of evaluation should be requested from persons who know the applicant well, who understand the academic and professional demands, and have had the opportunity to evaluate the applicant's personal qualities and potential as a professional person. The evaluator should be willing to write a thorough, comprehensive letter in the candidate's behalf.

Interviews may be requested, as deemed necessary, by the Dean and Admissions Committee to obtain additional information. The Dean and Admissions Committee may require additional evaluation procedures for selecting candidates for admission.

The School has an integrated curriculum which tends to prevent veterinary medical students of other universities from transferring into the School of Veterinary Medicine program at the University of California, Davis.

COLORADO STATE UNIVERSITY
School of Veterinary Medicine
  and Biomedical Sciences
Fort Collins, Colorado 80521

The professional School of Veterinary Medicine was established in 1907 with entrance requirements of 15 units of high school work. In 1932 the requirements were increased to graduation from an accredited high school, plus one year of pre-veterinary college work. Requirements were further increased in 1949 to two years of college and again, in 1972, increased to three years of pre-professional training to meet the minimum admission standards.

From 1907 through 1912 the professional curriculum took three years to complete; from 1913 on, four years were required for completion of the professional degree. The number of applicants to study veterinary medicine now far exceeds the ninety-four admitted to the freshman class each year. Selection is on a competitive basis for the most highly qualified.

Admission Requirements

Admission to the professional veterinary medicine program at Colorado State University (CSU) is restricted to students who either qualify for Colorado instate tuition or who are eligible for certification by a cooperating member state of the Western Interstate Commission for Higher Education (WICHE): Alaska, Arizona, Hawaii, Montana, Nevada, New Mexico, Utah, and Wyoming.

At least seven years of college work are required to obtain the degree, Doctor of Veterinary Medicine. The work is divided into a minimum of three years of pre-professional studies and, after acceptance into the professional program, four years of study.

At least 96 semester credits of acceptable college work are required for admission. Pre-professional courses may be taken at CSU or any nationally accredited junior college, college, or university.

The pre-professional curriculum serves two basic functions; it prepares students for application to the professional curriculum, and it provides a degree-oriented program in the health sciences and related fields for those who do not enter the professional veterinary program. Students are encouraged to pursue a bachelor's degree while completing the pre-professional requirements since it is a prime opportunity for them to broaden their education in fields contributing to careers and personal interests.

Credits obtained during the pre-professional curriculum may be applied toward a bachelor of science degree with a major in veterinary science only by those students who are accepted into the professional program. Veterinary science degree candidates must comply with the all-University requirments for graduation.

The non-academic requirements for admission consist of the applicant's character; achievements (i.e. leadership ability, as exemplified by participation in constructive activities outside formal academic areas); background and experience (working with livestock, laboratory animals, pets, and zoo animals); references (statements from employers, supervisors, or others who are familiar with the student's background and can testify to the applicant's character, experience, and knowledge); length of domicile in the state from which the applicant is applying; commitment, motivation, responsibility, and maturity (as evidenced by the quality and extent of undergraduate academic work and extracurricular activities); communicative skills; and familiarity with the many facets of the veterinary profession.

CORNELL UNIVERSITY
New York State College
  of Veterinary Medicine
Ithaca, New York 14850

Authorized by act of the legislature in 1894 and established in 1896, the College of Veterinary medicine is state supported but administered by the trustees of Cornell University, a private corporation.

The first class graduated in 1897. Prior to the formation of the veterinary college, Dr. James Law was professor of veterinary science at Cornell from 1868, when the University was founded. Under him, four men qualified for, and received the BVS degree.

Admission Requirements

Although the largest percentage of students admitted to the College of Veterinary Medicine are residents of New York State, a limited number of well-qualified non-resident applicants are also accepted. Candidates who feel their academic and other qualifications are outstanding are urged to apply, regardless of residency.

Admission to the New York State College of Veterinary Medicine requires a normal minimum of three years preparation in an accredited college or university. In exceptional cases, outstanding students who have completed all of the prerequisites in two years of undergraduate education may be considered for admission. This preparation does not have to be completed in a specialized college or in a designated pre-veterinary program. It is recommended that potential candidates seek an institution that offers the prerequisite courses as part of a baccalaureate program, has rigorous entrance requirements, and a national reputation for academic excellence. Because of limitations in class size, competition for admission is keen. Therefore, every candidate should have secondary career objectives. The best preparation for the study of veterinary medicine is to fulfill all entrance requirements while attaining excellence in the preparation for an alternate career.

Grades are not the sole criteria for admission, although it is desirable that the applicant have at least a 3.0 (4.0 scale) grade point average for all post-secondary academic work, and in particular, for the prerequisite courses when they are considered separately. Since it is impossible to evaluate honors, pass-fail, and S-U grading systems, it is necessary to obtain a letter grade for all of the prerequisite courses and have these grades certified by the registrar at the applicant's undergraduate institution.

The Graduate Record Examination (GRE) is a requirement for admission consideration. Arrangements should be made to the GRE no later than October of the year before desired matriculation.

By January 1 of the year in which the applicant seeks to matriculate, he or she must have fulfilled one of the two animal practice requirements. The two areas are the small animal practice and the large animal practice experiences. It is recommended that successful applicants fulfill both requirements before matriculation. Both requirements must be fulfilled before the third-year of registration at the College.

Only animal experience obtained after the age of fifteen will be acceptable. It is not possible for the College to furnish a list of potential employers. The applicant must pursue this on his own.

Clarification of the general appropriateness of work experience in satisfying the requirement may be obtained by submitting a detailed description of the work situation to the Office of Admissions in advance of actual application.

The following are the written requirements needed in addition to the basic application forms.

Essay on Aspirations for Veterinary Medicine

      An Animal Practice Essay
      Employer Evaluation Forms
      Evaluation from Faculty Advisor
      Letters of Recommendation

    Other factors to be considered when evaluating an applicant would be experience, knowledge, and achievements in extracurricular activites and matters unrelated to veterinary medicine. Ideally, the well-rounded person has accomplishments outside of the professional realm. Therefore, the committee evaluates the depth and breadth of achievement in extracurricular activities, community service, hobbies, and non-academic interests of all varieties.

    Aside from all the mentioned requirements, the committee endeavors to select candidates of high integrity, reliability, maturity and determination. It is important that professional people have excellent oral and written communicative skills, poise and leadership abilities, and have a talent for getting along with people.

UNIVERSITY OF FLORIDA
College of Veterinary Medicine
Gainesville, Florida 32601

In 1965 the Florida Legislature authorized the establishment of a College of Veterinary Medicine at the University of Florida. Funds for preliminary planning were appropriated in 1969 and 1970. A University advisory committee recommended that the instructional activities be developed, organized, and budgeted as a component of the University's J. Hillis Miller Health Center, and that the programs of the College concerned with extension and research on livestock and poultry diseases be developed and budgeted as part of the Institute of Food and Agricultural Sciences.

On April 1, 1971, a dean was appointed. At this time, an active planning program for the College was initiated.

Admission Requirements

Applicants are limited to residents of Florida and the Southern Regional Education Board (SREB) compact states.

All applicants to the professional curriculum must present a minimum of 120 quarter hours (80 semester hours) of college level course work, exclusive of courses in physical education and military training. Credit for the College Level Examination Program (CLEP) is acceptable at the level prescribed by the University of Florida.

Pre-veterinary requirements may be completed at any accredited two or four year college or university offering courses of content similar to those described in the University Record of the University of Florida, Gainesville. This study plan is designed to provide the educational basis that future veterinarians must have to satisfactorily meet the demands of the professional curriculum

Scholastic achievement will be measured by performance in the pre-professional courses. A student must have a grade point average of a least 2.75 on required pre-professional courses determined on an A=4.0 basis in order to be considered for admission. A grade of less than C in a required course will not be acceptable.

Successful completion of pre-veterinary requirements does not carry assurance that the student will be admitted to the College for training in veterinary medicine. Students are encouraged to complete courses leading to a baccalaureate degree.

Eligible candidates will be interviewed by members of the Faculty Committee on Admissions and will be carefully screened to assure that they are properly motivated, are equal to the rigorous course of professional study, and are competent to meet the performance demands of a professional career. Letters of reference will be requested from persons familiar with the applicant. There is no specific requirement for work experience with animals in any special field of the profession; however, applicants should have more than a general familiarity with animals and with the veterinary medical profession.

The privilege of matriculation may be denied any student whose mental or physical condition, as determined by a physician, is not considered satisfactory for the study of veterinary medicine.

An age limit has not been established for selection of candidates to entering classes. However, the number of productive years remaining in the anticipated life of an individual following graduation will be given consideration. Concern may be expressed about the motivation of an applicant desiring to abandon an established career to enter the College of Veterinary Medicine. Preference may be given to applicants who have shown a long standing fundamental interest in veterinary medicine.

Since new knowledge, especially in the sciences, is accruing at a phenomenal rate, it is recommended that all required science courses be completed within six calendar years immediately prior to application.

UNIVERSITY OF GEORGIA
College of Veterinary Medicine
Athens, Georgia 30601

A Division of Veterinary Medicine existed in the Georgia College of Agriculture from 1918-33. This unit granted 76 DVM degrees.

In 1946, a School of Veterinary Medicine was established by the Board of Regents of the University System of Georgia. The first class of students was admitted that fall and first year classes were taught in the College of Agriculture. Officially, the School of Veterinary Medicine became a separate unit in July, 1947. Also in that year a dean was appointed, and a new physical plant was begun.

In 1948, the School of Veterinary Medicine entered into a compact agreement with the states of Maryland, North Carolina, South Carolina, and Virginia. This compact called for, among other things, preferential consideration of applicants from those states in exchange for partial financial support of accepted students. This arrangement is still in effect.

The name was changed from School to College of Veterinary Medicine in 1970 by the Board of Regents. This was in recognition of the diversity of the overall program, including well-developed programs in undergraduate, professional and graduate study.

Admission Requirements

Application is open to legal residents of Georgia, North Carolina, South Carolina, Maryland and Virginia.

To qualify for admission to the University of Georgia College of Veterinary Medicine, a student must have acquired at least 90 quarter hours or 60 semester hours of college credit by the end of the spring quarter before fall matriculation at the College.

A student may complete the minimum required

courses while pursuing a pre-veterinary curriculum or while pursuing any other degree program of his or her choice at any accredited college or university. Because more applicants do not gain acceptance to the College than do, the College urges each applicant to pursue an alternate degree program while satisfying the course requirements for admission.

To be eligible for application, a student's cumulative grade point average on all college work completed within the last eight years must be at least 2.70 on a 4.0 grading system.

Each applicant will be required to take the Graduate Record Examination (GRE), including the Advanced Biology section, and the Veterinary Aptitude Test.

In addition to an applicant's academic performance, the Admissions Committee considers the previous activities and achievements, the knowledge and experience with animals, farm background, knowledge of veterinary medicine as a profession, letters of recommendation, and the applicant's narrative statement of purpose. Each applicant's performance in these areas is carefully evaluated. Preference is given to long-term residents of the contract states.

State officials who may be contacted for application forms and interview dates are:

Maryland
    Pre-veterinary Advisor
    Department of Veterinary Science
    College of Agriculture
    University of Maryland
    College Park, Maryland   20742

Virginia
    State Council of Higher Education
    700 Fidelity Building
    9th and Main Sts.
    Richmond, Virginia   23219

South Carolina
    Pre-veterinary Advisor
    Department of Poultry Science
    College of Agriculture and Biological Science
    Clemson University
    Clemson, South Carolina 29631

Georgia
    Associate Dean for Academic Affairs
    College of Veterinary Medicine
    University of Georgia
    Athens, Georgia 30602

UNIVERSITY OF ILLINOIS
College of Veterinary Medicine
Urbana, Illinois 61801

Although veterinary science courses have been offered in the College of Agriculture since 1870, the College of Veterinary Medicine was not established until 1944.

A four-story basic science building was completed in 1952, a large animal clinic in 1955. Other facilities include the small animal clinic, the diagnostic laboratory and the 80 acre veterinary research farm. The Veterinary Medical Research Building was completed in 1962, and an addition to the Diagnostic and Research annex was finished in 1965. The facilities for the College also include a new Veterinary Medicine Animal Clinic and Hospital complex at the College's relocation site. A new Basic Science Building for the relocation site is presently in the active planning stage.

Admission Requirements

Preference in admission is given to residents of Illinois; a limited number of non-residents with superior qualifications may be admitted. Non-residents offered admission will usually be from states that have no veterinary college or contractual agreement with a college of veterinary medicine in another state.

High school students interested in pursuing a career in veterinary medicine should complete courses in biology, chemistry, physics, and mathematics (through trigonometry), along with other courses required for graduation. Since admission requirements to pre-professional programs vary from college to college, high school students are urged to consult admission brochures of collegiate institutions that they may have under consideration.

The pre-professional program must include a

minimum of 60 semester hours (90 quarter hours) of college-level course work, exclusive of courses in physical education and military training. The courses are to be equivalent to those recommended for students majoring in biological sciences. It is strongly recommended that the science courses not be taken on a pass/fail option.

Pre-professional course requirements can be completed at most collegiate institutions. Students wishing to complete pre-professional requirements on the Urbana-Champaign campus of the University of Illinois may do so within a variety of curricula in either the College of Agriculture or the College of Liberal Arts and Sciences. Information regarding admission requirements to pre-professional programs offered on the Urbana-Champaign campus may be obtained by writing the Office of Admission and Records.

The Committee on Admission to the College of Veterinary Medicine will consider an application only if the applicant presents a minimum cumulative grade point average of 3.5 (3.0=C) at the end of the fall term preceding the desired date of admission. The applicant must also complete the 60 semester hours of pre-professional course requirements by the date of desired admission.

Completion of the minimum academic requirements does not guarantee admission to the professional curriculum.

Each applicant must provide official scores of his or her performance on the Veterinary Aptitude Test.

Three letters of recommendation are required from persons who can evaluate the applicant's experience and ability relating to professional and scientific study. Two letters should be from college instructors or academic advisors. A letter from a practicing veterinarian is considered highly desirable.

Applicants are expected to demonstrate potential for contribution to and advancement of the profession. An interview may be requested by the Committee as a means of supplementing information obtained from the materials submitted. Because of the physical demands of the veterinary profession and the program, a minimum amount of physical capability is required of all applicants admitted to the program. The Committee does not consider race, religion, national origin, sex or age in making its selections.

Applicants are ranked on the basis of a 100 point scale, with allocation of points distributed among the following criteria:

A) Objective Measures of Academic Performance - 70 points from grade point averages determined from official college transcripts and from Veterinary Aptitude Test VAT results. The cumulative grade point, science grade point, and total number of graded science hours completed, in addition to the score earned on the VAT will most likely be used to allocate these points.

B) Subjective Measures - Personal - 30 points allocated by the College Admission Advisory Committee on the basis of information submitted with the application and letters of recommendation indicating the applicant's knowledge of, motivation toward, and experience with the veterinary profession; evidence of leadership; initiative; and responsibility; animal contact and experience; extracurricular factors influencing personal growth.

C) Bonus Points - 2 bonus points will be assigned to veterans who have completed one or more years of active duty. Up to eight bonus points may be given to applicants for ancillary factors that have influenced academic performance: course loads (more credit for consistently heavy loads); improved trend in academic performance (benefit given for significant improvement following a "poor start"); course or course sequence quality (fulfilling a requirement with courses known for greater difficulty receives more credit).

Because of limitations in facilities and the

amount of support available to the College of Veterinary Medicine, the number of students who enter the professional curriculum each year must be restricted. In most recent years, there have been approximately 500 qualified applicants seeking the 86 spaces which have been funded for those years. The mean grade point average of the applicants selected has been slightly above the 4.50 (A=5.0) level, and the mean number of pre-professional hours completed has been near the 120 semester hour level.

IOWA STATE UNIVERSITY
College of Veterinary Medicine
Ames, Iowa 50010

Authorized in 1877, and established in 1879, the College of Veterinary Medicine of Iowa State University had its origin in the combined course in agriculture and veterinary medicine previously given at the College. At first, the entrance requirements were examinations in specified subjects; beginning in 1911, graduation from an approved high school was required. In 1931, one year of prescribed college work was added and, in 1949, two years of prescribed college work (90 quarter credits or 60 semester credits) were required for admission.

From 1879 to 1887, the professional curriculum covered two years, and was then increased to three years. In 1903, the course was extended to four years, the school being the first in this respect among American veterinary colleges.

The first class graduated in 1880, and consisted of five men who had had considerable advanced training and were given their degree after one year.

In considering applicants for admission to the College of Veterinary Medicine, preference is given to residents of Iowa and approved residents of states having contracts with Iowa State University for educating veterinary medical students. This is waived for minorities.

High school students contemplating careers in veterinary medicine should take the college preparatory program offered to those interested in biological sciences. A strong high school background in mathematics and the physical sciences, especially chemistry, is of value to the college student. High school students planning to enter Iowa State in the fall following graduation should apply at the beginning of their senior year. Persons planning to enter ISU other than fall quarter should apply at least six months in advance of the anticipated entry date. There is no limit to the number of academically qualified students who will be admitted to the pre-veterinary programs of the University. Admittance to the pre-veterinary programs does not imply admittance to the professional curriculum, the latter being limited and on a selective basis.

To become a veterinarian one must complete a prescribed program as a pre-veterinary college student and four years of study in the College of Veterinary Medicine. Iowa State University pre-veterinary students may enroll in either the College of Sciences and Humanities or in the College of Agriculture, depending upon their alternate educational goals.

Applicants for admission the the College of Veterinary Medicine for the fall quarter must have attended a regionally accredited college or university and received a bachelor's degree, or completed three years of a curriculum qualifying him or her to receive the bachelor's degree while pursuing the veterinary degree, or completed three years of a baccalaureate program meeting the general education requirements of the college attended. The student must have earned at least 144 quarter (96) semester credits.

Credits will normally be earned on the traditional four-letter grading system with "A" as the highest grade and "D" as the lowest passing grade. However, credits earned by the test-out program in accordance with the regulations relating to this procedure at Iowa State University are also acceptable. Credits in the preceding specified courses will not be accepted if earned under the Pass- Not Pass grading system or similar options. All students just have completed at least 90 quarter (60 semester) credits prior to filing an application for admission to the College of Veterinary Medicine.

Pre-professional college credits must average at least 2.50 on a 4.0 marking system for the application to be accepted. The preceding scholastic requirements are minimum and do not assure admission even though these requirements have been fulfilled.

Admission to the College of Veterinary Medicine is on a competitive and selective basis. Scholastic performance in pre-professional courses, aptitude and personal development are given consideration in the selection of candidates. Since a solid foundation in the sciences is basis to success in veterinary medicine, considerable attention is given in the admission process to applicants' grades in those areas. Consideration for admission to the College of Veterinary Medicine is administered equally to all without regard to race, color, creed, sex, national origin, disability, or age. Admission is granted annually at the beginning of the fall quarter only, with enrollment limited to 120 students per class.

KANSAS STATE UNIVERSITY
College of Veterinary Medicine
Manhattan, Kansas 66502

The curriculum leading to the degree, Doctor of Veterinary Medicine, was established at Kansas State effective in 1905. However, beginning in 1886, courses were offered to students enrolled in Agriculture, but not for veterinary degree credit. At first, the school was known as the Department of Veterinary Medicine; it became the Division of Veterinary Medicine in 1919, and in 1943 the name Division was changed to School. In 1963 it was designated a full College.

Admission Requirements

Selection for admission to the professional program in veterinary medicine will be on individual merit from qualified applicants who are graduates of Kansas high schools, and who together with their parents are residents of Kansas, and have been residents for at least three years immediately prior to first semester enrollment of the year for which they are applying; or who have been wholly independent residents of Kansas for five years immediately prior to first semester enrollment of the year for which they are applying. After Kansans are selected, non-residents from states with which Kansas State has a contract for reimbursement will be selected. Currently, contracts are in effect with Arizona, Arkansas, Hawaii, Nebraska, Nevada, New Jersey, New Mexico, North Dakota, Oregon, Puerto Rico, South Dakota, Utah, and Wyoming.

For the pre-veterinary medical curriculum, the high school graduate should have a strong academic record, excellent ACT scores, and have completed one and one-half units of algebra and one unit of plane geometry. Other high school subjects which are highly recommended for a pre-veterinary medical student are chemistry, mathematics, physics and biology. A strong background in oral and written communications is also desirable.

Enrollment in the College of Veterinary Medicine is limited to 100 well-qualified students after a minimum of two years of college work which includes the required 64 semester hours of pre-veterinary medical courses. The 100 students are selected from more than 1000 applicants, with preference given to Kansans. A student must have at least a 3.0 (A=4.0) average over the pre-professional requirements and the last 45 hours of undergraduate college work in order to be interviewed for selection. Non-residents from contract states need to meet the same scholastic requirements to receive an application for the professional curriculum and consideration for selection.

Only those students who can complete the required 64 semester hours of pre-veterinary medical training by the end of the spring term in the year in which they are seeking admission will be considered for admission to the professional curriculum of veterinary medicine.

Personal interviews are required of all students under consideration. Selection is based upon academic achievement and professional potential as determined by the interview with the admissions committee. In recent years the majority of the successful candidates have had more than four years of pre-veterinary work.

Inquiries for further specific information about veterinary medicine are welcome.

Address them to:

Assistant Dean
College of Veterinary Medicine
Veterinary Medical Teaching Building
Kansas State University
Manhattan, Kansas 66506.

LOUISIANA STATE UNIVERSITY
School of Veterinary Medicine
Baton Rouge, Louisiana   70803

The School of Veterinary Medicine was established in 1962 and again in 1967 by resolution of the LSU Board of Supervisors, and it was authorized in 1968 through action of the Louisiana State Legislature. The School, the only new program in veterinary medicine to receive federal support for establishment under the Health Professions Educational Assistance Program, BHME, NIH, is one of the new multi-state participations to be added to the Southern Region.

The first entering class of 36 students was selected in August, 1973, and instruction in veterinary medicine began on January 3, 1974.

The School participates in the Southern Regional Education Board's program for education in veterinary medicine. Training contracts negotiated through SREB provide a limited number of entering spaces for candidates from Arkansas and West Virginia.

Pre-veterinary requirements may be completed at Louisiana State University or at any accredited college or university offereing courses of the content and quality of those prescribed in the LSU catalogue.

The minimum requirements, 69 semester hours of credit (inclusive of nine hours of elective courses) may be completed in two years. Admission to, or successful completion of the pre-veterinary curriculum does not carry assurance that the student will be admitted to the School for participation in the professional program.

The two-year pre-veterinary curriculum at LSU is summarized in the catalogue. It is administered by the College of Agriculture. Students who enroll in the pre-professional curriculum at accredited institutions other than Louisiana State University must determine that courses taken conform in content and quality to descriptions contained in the latest

LSU catalogue.

Official transcripts of previous works are examined to determine scholastic achievement and three grade-point averages are calculated and evaluated:
- A) the pre-professional grade point average determined from grades received in all required work completed in the prescribed pre-professional curriculum;
- B) the science grade point average - determined from grades received in prescribed science courses (44 of the 69 semester credit hours), i.e. mathematics, biology, chemistry and physics, genetics, etc.; and
- C) the last 45 semester credit hours grade point average - this average is derived from grades earned in courses of substantive quality taken during the last three semesters or equivalent. Credits earned in graduate study are included in the GPA determination.

New knowledge, especially in the sciences, is occurring at a phenomenal rate and the records of students who have completed the pre-professional requirements several years prior to application will be carefully scrutinized. All required science courses should be completed within six calendar years immediately prior to application.

The scores received from the School and College Ability Test (SCAT) are included in the objective evaluation.

Louisiana applicants must satisfy all residency requirements as defined in University regulations, including the one-year time requirement, prior to the February 15 application deadline. Determination of residency status and evaluation of each applicant's record in the pre-professional curriculum is made in accordance with the procedure in force in the Office of Admissions, LSU, Baton Rouge. Each state participating under the SREB program maintains a counseling service for students desiring admission to the LSU School of Veterinary Medicine. Interested persons should contact their respective program coordinators as early as possible for information concerning requirements for admission, for application, and for residency. Applicants from contract states must be certified as having residency or citizenship established as required by the contract state by the date of the application deadline. The application submission deadline for regional students is February 1 of the calendar year in which admission is sought.

Eligible candidates are interviewed by members of the Faculty Committee on Admissions, and are carefully selected to make sure they are properly motivated, are equal to the rigorous course of professional study, and are competent to meet the performance demands of a professional career. There is no minimum requirement for work experience with animals or for work experience in some field of the profession. In the judgement of the Committee, applicants should have more than a general familiarity with animals, and with the veterinary medical profession. The significance of applicant experience in these areas is determined from the credentials presented with the application and from specifics obtained through the interview.

Motivation, maturity, attitude, interest and certain qualities of character will be evaluated for all qualified candidates, along with work experience. familiarity with animals and reference information submitted in support of the application. These qualities are considered by members of the Admissions Committee during application review and during the candidate interview.

MICHIGAN STATE UNIVERSITY
College of Veterinary Medicine
East Lansing, Michigan 48823

Courses in veterinary science had been taught at East Lansing since 1878 by what was then called Michigan Agricultural College. In 1909 the Michigan legislature authorized a complete program leading to the DVM degree, which the governing board established in 1910 as a four-year curriculum under a Division of Veterinary Science. The name was changed to School of Veterinary Medicine in 1955 when the parent institution became Michigan State University.

At first, the entrance requirement was graduation from high school. In 1935, one year of pre-veterinary college work was added. Beginning in 1949, two years of pre-professional training was required for admission. At present, at least 85 quarter credits, including certain prescribed courses, are required for admission.

Admission Requirements

Applicants are considered for admission with priority given to citizens of the United States who are residents of the State of Michigan. Because Michigan State University is a public tax-assisted institution, it is obligated to give admission priority to Michigan residents as defined by Michigan State University for fee purposes.

A limited number of spaces (approximately 10 percent) are expected to be available for highly qualified out-of-state residents. For these spaces, consideration priority is expected to be as follows:
 A) Michigan State University students who are residents of states not having a veterinary school or participating in the Southern Regional Education Board, or the Western Interstate Commission for Higher Education.

B) Non-Michigan State University students who are residents of states not having a veterinary school or participating in SREB or WICHE.
C) Residents of states having a veterinary school or participating in SREB or WICHE.
D) Citizens of foreign countries.

Note that particularly applicants in category "B" from states having contracts and/or agreements for a substantial number of spaces, and in categories "C" and "D" should not expect serious consideration.

Pre-professional courses must be completed before admission to the professional program. (College credits must be earned for required pre-veterinary science courses listed below: biochemistry, biology, chemistry, mathematics, physics, and zoology). Because the Selection Committee is unable to determine levels of competency achieved in subject matter covered in courses graded "credit", "pass", "satisfactory" etc., it is advisable to take pre-professional courses on a letter or numerical grade basis.

These pre-professional course requirements may be completed at Michigan State University in a two-year program or, alternatively, in conjunction with a four-year degree program (i.e. biological science, zoology, animal husbandry, medical technology, microbiology, and public health etc.)

While enrollment in the pre-veterinary program at Michigan State is not limited, enrollment in the professional program is limited to 115 students accepted per year.

Students interested in entering Michigan State University for pre-veterinary study should write for admission and financial aid information to:

Office of Admissions and Scholarships
250 John A. Hannah Administration Building
East Lansing, Michigan 48824.

The following factors are considered by the Selection Committee in determining an applicant's relative competitive position:
- cumulative grade point average (emphasis on the undergraduate record)
- grade point average for required pre-veterinary science courses
- average credit load per term
- total credits completed
- Veterinary Aptitude Test score.

The following are additional factors considered by the Selection Committee in determining an applicant's relative competitive position:
- interview score
- veterinary exposure score
- animal exposure score
- activities and achievements of the applicant
- evidence of communication skills.

Applications and admission information may be obtained from:

Admissions Office
College of Veterinary Medicine
Michigan State University
East Lansing, Michigan 48824.

THE UNIVERSITY OF MINNESOTA
College of Veterinary Medicine
St. Paul, Minnesota 55101

    The College of Veterinary Medicine at the University of Minnesota was established by the 1947 Legislature and the University Board of Regents as a School of Veterinary Medicine. On July 1, 1957 the Board of Regents established it as a College of Veterinary Medicine with the same administrative status as the other professional colleges in the University. Since its inception in 1947, the College has continually expanded its facilities for teaching, research, and public service. The 1971 Legislature appropriated funds for further expansion of the College. Construction of a new building (Phase I of a planned building expansion program) was completed in fall, 1975, and the building was occupied in January, 1976. This facility houses portions of both basic science and clinical science facilities.

    The College of Veterinary Medicine at the University of Minnesota traditionally has served as a regional facility, providing educational opportunities for residents of neighboring states, viz., North Dakota, South Dakota, and Wisconsin, as well as for Minnesotans. In the recent past, compacts have been made with Wisconsin, North Dakota, and Nebraska to enable guaranteed numbers of their residents to attend the College at resident tuition rates, with the home state contributing to the cost of the students' education. As total enrollment increases beyond the 80 currently admitted, the College plans to increase the number of students accepted.

    The Committee on Admissions, in selecting applicants, gives first priority to Minnesota residents and to residents of states with which contractual or reciprocity agreements exist. Currently, these states include Nebraska, North Dakota, and Wisconsin. This priority applies to all but minority applicants.

In order to increase the pool of minority applicants, the Committee on Admissions waives the residency preference when considering racial/ethnic minorities. Such students are encouraged to contact the Coordinator of Minority Recruitment in the Office of Professional and Undergraduate Education.

Admission Requirements

Applicants for admission to the University of Minnesota College of Veterinary Medicine are ranked on the basis of a 100 point scale with the allocation of points distributed among the areas of evaluation as follows:
- A) Objective Measures of Education Background 70 points
    1. grade point average - minimum course requirements - 30 points
    2. most recent cumulative grade point average - most recent terms, and going back to include a minimum of 60 quarter (45 semester) credits of letter grade in undergraduate and/or graduate courses - 12 points
    3. Graduate Record Examination - 10 points
    4. Veterinary Aptitude Test - 10 points
    5. amount of collegiate experience - 8 points
- B) Subjective Measures - Personal Experience - 30 points
    1. maturity and reliability - employment experiences and responsibilities, ability to communicate with others, experiences suggesting leadership, extracurricular activities, credit load and the amount of time devoted to employment and other activities while enrolled in college 15 points.

Veterinary Medicine application packets should be requested from the Office of Admissions and Records.

MISSISSIPPI STATE UNIVERSITY
College of Veterinary Medicine
Mississippi State, Mississippi   39762

The Mississippi College of Veterinary Medicine was established by an act of the Legislature on March 12, 1974. Dr. James G. Miller was named to be the First Dean of the College.

The College program was planned by a group of veterinary educators representing many of the colleges of veterinary medicine, regulatory medicine, and private practice.

Architectural plans for the College were approved by the 1976 Legislature and $12,500,000 appropriated for construction of a teaching hospital.

The initial faculty was recruited from twelve of the established colleges of veterinary medicine in the United States and Canada.

The College achieved "Reasonable Expectation of Accreditation" from the AVMA Council on Education in 1977.

The first professional class in the DVM program was admitted in May of 1977.

Admission Requirements

Applicants who meet the requirements for the College of Veterinary Medicine will be accorded an evaluation based on a two phase program. The applicants will receive points for both academic and non-academic credentials. At the completion of the first phase, the combined totals of these criteria will be computed and finalists will be invited to participate in a second state evaluation process. The remainder will receive, upon their request, counseling relevant to their possible future academic programs.

The breakdown of the evaluation follows.

Phase I

The evaluation of the applicants is based on four primary factors:
1. academic record
2. applicant's statement and answers to application questions
3. applicant's familiarity with animal behavior and animal handling skills
4. applicant interview.

In the first phase, the academic record of the potential candidate will receive considerable weight 1200 points. The applicant's overall GPA, grades received in science courses, required courses, and the last two semesters are included in those factors evaluated. The applicant's non-academic record will receive 900 points of the total 2100 points allocated to Phase I.

The first phase interview is worth 400 points, and will be conducted at the College of Veterinary Medicine, Mississippi State University, and will include an assessment of the candidate's potential for serving the public in the field of veterinary medicine. All interviewers will have undergone specific training in interviewing techniques. A period of approximately 45 minutes will be allocated for each candidate, during which time they will be evaluated for such characteristics as communication skills, self-determination, professionalism and adaptability.

Each interviewer will rate the candidate numerically. An average of the two ratings will constitute the interview score.

Arrangements will be made to send a team of interviewers to off-campus areas in those cases where numbers and logistics warrant such consideration.

Application statement and responses are worth 250 points. The candidate's statement of his reasons for wanting to enter the College of Veterinary Medicine and responses concerning other issues will be evaluated,

125 points for communication skills (evaluated by the English Department), and 125 points for relevant content (evaluated by the Veterinary Faculty). Members of the faculty will read the statement and rate the content. An average of the Faculty ratings plus the rating by the English Department will consitute the total evaluation.

Animal contact is worth 250 points. Experience with animals and animal handling is considered to be an important characteristic.

Phase II

The second phase evaluation represents an in-depth assessment of the applicant's non-academic characteristics which are stressed in contrast to the weighing of academic characteristics in Phase I.

In Phase II, the student will participate in a three-day assessment and orientation session in small groups. Students are assigned to mentors who serve as guides and advisors throughout the procedure. A major effort is made to portray the nature, demands, and characteristics of undergraduate life in the veterinary college. It is important that the student be aware of the demands made on his or her personal and financial resources before he or she and the College make a commitment to embark on the four year program.

Final assessment of the applicant will be based on scores accumulated in both academic (300) and non-academic (900) scales plotted on a two-dimensional scattergram from which the class will be selected.

Applicants will participate in the following activities during Phase II of the admission procedure. These activities will be scheduled in a three-day assessment and orientation session held at the College of Veterinary Medicine on the campus at Mississippi State University.
    1. Communication Profile (200 points)
        Veterinary medical practice requires competence in the spoken and written language.

Reading and comprehension skills are an integral part of the veterinarian's lifelong study. One aspect of the admission process is the evaluation of the communication skills of the applicant. This evaluation will examine the applicant's ability to read with understanding and to discriminate between the meanings of vocabulary words.

2. Interviews (400 points)
   This will be an in-depth discussion with the applicant utilizing some of the same factors as in Phase I; i.e. communication skills, self-determination, professionalism, and adaptability. However, the interview inquiries will deal with the immediate experiences of the three-day assessment and orientation sessions. Interviews will be conducted by interview teams composed of faculty and non-faculty members using individual interview rating forms.

3. Animal Handling (250 points)
   This evaluation is intended to assess the applicant's awareness and rapport with different animal species. It will involve safe handling procedures and normal behavioral characteristics of animals. These procedures will include, but may not be limited to, restraint, haltering, and recording observations of the animal, estimating weights, determining sex, and identifying breeds. The scoring of this activity will not necessarily be based on the applicant's knowledge and ability in handling the different animal species, but rather upon his or her approach to the problem in dealing with unfamiliar situations, if that is the case.

4. Academic Profile (300 points)
The academic profile of the applicant will be part of the evaluation in the second phase. However, during Phase II less weight will be given to the academic characteristics of the applicant.

5. Log Book Observations (50 points)
A log book will be supplied to each applicant for recording observations and reactions to the assessment and orientation sessions. The following activites will be reflected in the student's recorded responses:
    a. Typical Veterinary School Lecture - this experience is provided for the applicant's orientation to the didactic areas of the curriculum and its demands. Reference to the experience during the interview is likely.
    b. Film "Covenant" and Discussion - this film explores the professional career of veterinary medicine describing opportunities and competency demands of memberships in the profession. It will provide recent career background information for interviewing the applicant.
    c. Necropsy Demonstration and Film "Animal Heart Surgery" - the necropsy demonstration and film will provide direct and vicarious experience to the applicant of tasks commonly performed by veterinarians. Reactions of the applicant to these experiences may be basis for inquiries during the interview.
    d. Honor Code -professionalism demands adherence to a code of ethics and

its beginning can be found in most veterinary schools in this country in the form of an Honor Code. This is a program operated by the students and the College by which trust and faith is placed in each by his fellow students and faculty to uphold the standards of honesty and trustworthiness both in and outside the classroom. These concepts will be discussed and explained so that each potential veterinary student will understand what is expected of him when admitted into the professional curriculum.

    e. Dress Code - the professional student is expected to appear neat and clean at all times and to dress in an acceptable manner to suit the occassion. Dress is usually an outward manifestation of inner feelings. The dress code of this school will be presented and students accepted into the curriculum will be expected to live up to those standards.

6. Manipulative Coordination
The delivery of many veterinary practice skills requires a normal degree of manual coordination; i.e. minor surgery, suturing, taking of specimens for examination, etc. The valuative procedures are designed to assess the applicant's manipulative coordination which will be necessary to perform clinical procedures. Standardized measures of eye-hand coordination and veterinary oriented procedures will be utilized.

7. A preference inventory will be administered

to each applicant. The results will be
presented to the applicant as feedback for
counseling purposes and instructional purposes.

For information on application procedures, write
to the

Office of the Dean
Drawer V
Mississippi State University
Mississippi State, Mississippi 39762.

UNIVERSITY OF MISSOURI
College of Veterinary Medicine
Columbia, Missouri 65201

Veterinary Medicine at the University of Missouri at Columbia is based on the long-standing concern for livestock health in Missouri. The first instruction in veterinary medicine at UMC was offered in 1872.

Strong impetus was given to veterinary medicine at UMC by Dr. John W. Connaway, who became head of the Department of Veterinary Science in 1892. Dr. Connaway, in collaboration with Dr. Mark Francis of Texas, conducted the key research which lead to the solution of the problem of Texas fever. Dr. Connaway went on to direct the Hog Cholera vaccination program and serum production in Missouri. He was also a strong proponent for establishing a professional-level veterinary curriculum at UMC.

In 1946, the first students were admitted to the new professional program. In 1949, the Department of Veterinary Science became the School of Veterinary Medicine. The first class graduated in 1950. Starting in 1977, 72 students were admitted each year to the professional curriculum. The School became the College of Veterinary Medicine in 1974.

Admission Requirements

Since the UMC College of Veterinary Medicine is a state-supported instituion, and there are far more applicants each year than can be admitted, it has been necessary to establish the following priorities concerning admission.
1. First preference is extended to residents of Missouri.
2. Second-level consideration is usually extended to applicants from states without schools of veterinary medicine.
3. Third-level consideration is generally

granted to applicants from states with schools of veterinary medicine.
4. Out-of-state applicants should establish scholastic records of at least B+ (3.5 on a 4.0=A system) in order to receive serious consideration for admission.

There are no fixed requirements for the high school curriculum as preparation for the pre-professional course work. However, the student is wise to concentrate in three areas: mathematics, English, and communication skills, and some exposure to science. Actually, veterinary medicine may be considered an applied form of biological science. Therefore, it is probably wise for a student to take four years of math, four years of English, two years of biology, and as much chemistry and physics as is possible.

A minimum of two years of pre-professional study is required before a student may be admitted to the professional program leading to the Doctor of Veterinary Medicine (DVM) degree at the UMC College of Veterinary Medicine. Pre-veterinary medical requirements may be completed at any accredited college or university where the course work is offered.

Students interested in completing the pre-professional requirements at UMC should address inquiries to the Office of Admissions.

Admittance to the professional curriculum depends upon the approval of the Committee on Admissions and Scholarship for the College of Veterinary Medicine.

Students must complete at least 64 semester hours of college work by the end of the winter semester (spring quarter) of the year in which admission is sought. However, very few students are admitted with only the minimum number of credits (average of those admitted is usually over 100 semester hours). Therefore, students are encouraged to take concurrent course work which will satisfy a major at the bachelor's degree level. Since only 72 students are admitted each year into the veterinary curriculum, they are encouraged to pursue bachelor's degrees in areas in which they would like to work if they are not accepted into veterinary school.

A Missouri resident must have attained an accumulative grade point average of 2.5 (A=4.0) or better during pre-professional work in order to have an application accepted. While the minimum requirements for admission may be completed in two years of study, students admitted with only two years of pre-professional work are usually those with exceptionally good scholastic achievement records and aptitude scores.

After initial screening, the remaining applicants are also evaluated on the basis of their personal interviews (when required), experience, and personal references. The committee selects students with as many of the following characteristics as possible: reasonable judgement and common sense, moderately wide range of interests, some evidence of leadership ability, pleasing and alert personality, willingness to work for a worthwhile objective, and at least fair understanding of the scope of veterinary medicine.

THE OHIO STATE UNIVERSITY
College of Veterinary Medicine
Columbus, Ohio   43210

Established in 1885 as the School of Veterinary Medicine, Ohio State University made it the College of Veterinary Medicine in 1897. The school had its origin when the Board of Trustees of the University, realizing the proportion of the state's wealth which was invested in livestock and sensing the need for its adequate protection from contagious diseases, petitioned the legislature for the establishment of a veterinary college.

At first, the entrance requirements were either examinations in specified subjects, high school graduation, or a teacher's certificate. In 1906, the requirements were increased by examination in additional subjects, a high school diploma being accepted in lieu of examination for such required subjects as it included. In 1933, one year of pre-veterinary college work was required and, beginning with the academic year 1949-1950, two years.

Admission Requirements

In the selection of students, consideration will be given both residents and non-residents of the State of Ohio. Preference will be shown to highly qualified applicants between the ages of 20 and 28 years who are residents of the State of Ohio as determined by the rules set forth by the Ohio Board of Regents. Non-residents will be considered on a competitive basis from states with which The Ohio State University has a veterinary medical education agreement. The veterinary medical education agreement states include: Kentucky, Maryland, New Hampshire, New Jersey, North Carolina, Virginia, and West Virginia. Applicants from the agreement states should obtain details concerning admissions procedures from their respective State Office of Higher Education. Appointees must be citizens of the United States.

A student who is enrolled in the Ohio State University may complete the pre-professional course requirements in the College of Arts and Sciences, or in the College of Agriculture and Home Economics. Since it is not possible to accept all eligible applicants, alternate goals in standard BA and BS degree programs are urged for all veterinary medical pre-professional students.

Non-resident students enrolled at this university should be aware that the veterinary medical pre-professional course requirements for admission to The Ohio State University College of Veterinary Medicine do not always satisfy the veterinary medical pre-professional course requirements for admission to other colleges of veterinary medicine.

The Veterinary Aptitude Test is required of all applicants and should be taken after the end of the last term of the sophmore year in college. It is recommended that the student have credit for a basic year of biology, or zoology, general and organic chemistry, mathematics, and physics prior to taking the test.

Those qualified applicants with grade-point averages of 3.00 or above (based upon a system where 4.00=A) and earning a satisfactory score on the Veterinary Aptitude Test will be invited for an interview. All candidates are selected on a competitive basis considering grade-point average, VAT score, performance in required pre-professional science courses, and the average number of hours carried per term.

Each year there are a large number of candidates for admission to the College of Veterinary Medicine. Only those applicants whose pre-professional work in college is of superior quality may expect to be admitted. Many applicants must spend three years or more in pre-professional study before being admitted to the College of Veterinary Medicine.

Other factors which will be considered in the selection of students are written and verbal expression, personal evaluations, knowledge of the profession, experience with animals, veterinary medical work related experiences, and motivation.

OKLAHOMA STATE UNIVERSITY
College of Veterinary Medicine
Stillwater, Oklahoma 74074

Oklahoma Agricultural and Mechanical College and the Agricultural Experiment Station was established by an act of the First Territorial Legislature in 1890. The School of Veterinary Medicine was established in 1947.

The name of the College was changed to Oklahoma State University, and the School was changed to College in 1957.

From the beginning, the professional curriculum had covered four years of training in addition to the minimum two pre-professional years.

Admission Requirements

An applicant must be a legal resident of Oklahoma according to regulations governing pursuit of higher education in Oklahoma. Questions about residency should be directed to the registrar of Oklahoma State. He has final authority in matters of residency pertaining to Oklahoma State University.

As for secondary school preparation, English composition, public speaking, mathematics, general science, biology, chemistry, and physics are necessary. Generally, a student who has a basic interest in science and a high aptitude in mathematics has little difficulty meeting these academic requirements.

Those individuals applying for admission in the fall must satisfy all admission requirements by the end of the fall semester in which admission is desired. A student may complete the pre-professional curriculum in any accredited institution, but such courses and credits must be evaluated at Oklahoma State University before an applicant's eligibility is approved. Although only two years of pre-professional course work are required, most students admitted to the College of Veterinary Medicine have completed three to four years.

To be eligible to receive an application packet, an applicant must have a grade point average of at least 2.8 (A=4.0) in the specific required courses completed when the application packet is requested. A grade lower than "C" in a required course is not acceptable, and either the course must be repeated or a higher level course which has the approval of the Admissions Committee may be substituted. In either case, the hours and grade points of the repeated course(s) or substitute course(s) are added to those of the original course to arrive at the grade point average. Likewise, all hours attempted, whether passed or not, are calculated in the cumulative grade point average.

The Admissions Committee considers the weighted scores for Required Course GPA, Cumulative GPA, and SCAT total score.

The Admissions Committee also considers personal interview scores, letters of recommendation, and the applicant's handwritten personal statements concerning his or her interest in veterinary medicine.

All inquiries pertaining to admissions should be addressed to:

> College of Veterinary Medicine
> Attention: Admissions Secretary
> Oklahoma State University
> Stillwater, Oklahoma 74074.

UNIVERSITY OF PENNSYLVANIA
School of Veterinary Medicine
Philadelphia, Pennsylvania 19104

First proposed in 1807 by a member of the medical faculty at the University of Pennsylvania, the school was authorized by the Board of Trustees in 1878, established in 1883, and actually opened in 1884. This is the only school of the currently accredited veterinary colleges in the United States which had it origin in medicine rather than in agriculture.

At first, admission was by examination in specified subjects, or by high school certificate. In 1914, two years of high school were required for entrance and this was raised to four years in 1916. In 1936, one year of pre-veterinary college work was required and, in 1940, two years. Starting in 1970, the required minimum was increased to three years of pre-veterinary college work.

Admission Requirements

Any student who has fulfilled all of the requirements listed in the catalogue can apply to the school regardless of their state of legal residence. However, seventy percent of each entering class is selected from the Pennsylvania applicant pool, and most of the remaining seats are reserved for contract state residents. The contract states are all of the New England states except Massachusetts, plus New Jersey, Delaware, Maryland, and Puerto Rico.

The minimum educational requirements for admission to the School of Veterinary Medicine are, in all but exceptional circumstances, the satisfactory completion of three years study in a college or university accredited by the Association of American Colleges and Universities, or one of the regional accrediting associations. The three years of college study must total 90 semester credits (135 quarter credits) exclusive of animal husbandry subjects.

All applicants must submit to the School of Veterinary Medicine scores obtained on the Graduate Record Examination Aptitude Test (GRE).

The Committee on Admissions also considers the applicant's apparent familiarity with the profession and resultant sincerity of interest; recommendations of academic counselors; recommendations of veterinarians with whom the applicant has had work experience; character; personality and general fitness; and adaptability for a career in veterinary medicine.

Experience with some aspect of veterinary medicine is considered essential by the Admission Committee and should be documented. The applicant should request that letters of recommendation be forwarded to the Admissions Office for inclusion in the application file. All letters of recommendation will be acknowledged to the sender.

OREGON STATE UNIVERSITY
School of Veterinary Medicine
Corvallis, Oregon 97330

   Courses in veterinary science were among the subjects taught at Oregon State Agriculture College as early as 1892. In 1910, the Department of Veterinary Science was established within the School of Agriculture. In 1914, a veterinarian was employed, and the name of the Department was changed to Veterinary Medicine.
   In 1975, the State Legislature, responding to the need for more veterinarians in Oregon, and the need for increasing opportunities for Oregonians to study veterinary medicine, established the School of Veterinary Medicine at Oregon State University.

Admission Requirements

   A minimum of three years of college-level preparation is required before a student can be accepted for entry into the School of Veterinary Medicine. These years of instruction may be taken at any institution that has courses equivalent to those taught at Oregon State. The courses include studies in communications, arts and humanities, and social sciences as well as a major course of study in the physical and biological sciences.
   Completion of the general aptitude section of the Graduate Record Examination is also required. In addition to the academic requirements, the applicant must have been employed by, worked on a volunteer basis for, or by some other means gained significant contact with a graduate veterinarian.
   The OSU School of Veterinary Medicine has an agreement with the College of Veterinary Medicine at Washington State University, Pullman, and the University of Idaho, Moscow, for a cooperative program in veterinary medical education leading to the degree of

Doctor of Veterinary Medicine. This agreement, which created the WOI Program in Veterinary Medical Education, is unique in that students may receive instruction on three campuses.

Each year, twenty-eight residents of Oregon, and eight residents from the Western Regional Compact States (Alaska, Hawaii, Montana, Nevada, New Mexico, Utah, and Wyoming) will enter Oregon State University and take their first year of professional study on the Corvallis campus. The thirty-six Oregon-sponsored students will then transfer to Washington State University for their second and part of their third year of study. These students, at the end of April in their third year, will then transfer back to Oregon State University to complete their third year and to take their fourth and final year of instruction. Students may also elect to receive instruction during their fourth year at the Unversity of Idaho's Food Animal Referral Clinic at Caldwell, Idaho.

Oregon residents desiring additional information about veterinary medicine should write to:

> The Office of the Dean
> School of Veterinary Medicine
> Oregon State University
> Corvallis, Oregon 97331.

Residents from other states should write to

> The Office of Student Services
> College of Veterinary Medicine
> Washington State University
> Pullman, Washington 99164.

PURDUE UNIVERSITY
School of Veterinary Medicine
Lafayette, Indiana 47901

In 1957 the Indiana General Assembly authorized the establishment of the School of Veterinary Science and Medicine at Purdue University. The first class of fifty students was enrolled in 1959.

Prior to the establishment of the School, a Department of Veterinary Science had existed at Purdue University since 1887, primarily as a research and service department in the Purdue Agricultural Experiment Station. The research, extension, and diagnostic activities of this department have been retained in conjunction with the School of Veterinary Medicine.

Admission Requirements

Since enrollment is limited, first preference will be given to Indiana residents. There is limited admission of non-resident students and preference in this category is given to those who are residents of states not having veterinary medical schools.

If an individual expects to apply for admission to the professional degree program in the School of Veterinary Medicine, he or she must first complete a two-year pre-professional (or pre-veterinary) curriculum. The pre-veterinary curriculum at Purdue is offered in the School of Agriculture and the School of Science.

Students in one of the other schools of the University, having completed the required courses or their equivalents, are eligible to apply for admission to the professional program in the School of Veterinary Medicine. Since enrollment in the professional school is limited, completion of the pre-veterinary program does not insure admittance to the School of Veterinary Medicine. All courses required by the Admissions Committee and the Dean, including those in progress at the time of application, must be completed satisfactorily.

The following are also considered by the Admissions Committee for selection of students: maturity, character, and motivation. Animal experience and a reasonable acquaintance with the veterinary medical profession are highly desirable. Not all applicants are invited for interviews, but a personal interview is required for all applicants who are in the final pool from which the class will be selected.

UNIVERSITY OF TENNESSEE
College of Veterinary Medicine
Knoxville, Tennessee 37916

In 1974 the Tennessee Legislature authorized establishment of the College of Veterinary Medicine as a unit of the state-wide Institue of Agriculture of the University of Tennessee. Headquarters and principal facilities of the College are located on the Knoxville campus of the University. Satellite facilities for teaching and research are located at several other locations in the state.

The College has a unique administrative organization. The Department of Animal Science is jointly administered by the College of Veterinary Medicine and the College of Agriculture. The Department of Microbiology is jointly administered by the College of Veterinary Medicine and the College of Liberal Arts. Four other departments are administered exclusively by the College of Veterinary Medicine: Pathobiology, Enviormental Practice, Urban Practice, Rural Practice.

The first class was admitted in September, 1976.

Admission Requirements

Currently, applications are accepted only from residents of Tennessee. At some future, but as yet undetermined time, it is anticipated that a limited number of out-of-state residents may be admitted to the professional program.

A minimum of 115 quarter credits (or 78 semester credits) of college work must be completed before admission to the professional curriculum of the College of Veterinary Medicine.

All pre-veterinary requirements must be completed by the end of the spring term of the year in which the individual plans to enroll in the professional curriculum of the College of Veterinary Medicine.

Admission to the College of Veterinary Medicine

will be for the fall quarter of each year. Enrollment will be limited to that number of students for which a high quality education can be provided with available facilities and resources. Applicants to the College, therefore, will be screened carefully by a faculty committee.

Residency status may be determined, and forms for making application for admission may be obtained by writing to:

> Director of Admissions
> The University of Tennessee
> 305 Student Services Building
> Knoxville, Tennessee 37916.

TEXAS A & M UNIVERSITY
College of Veterinary Medicine
College Station, Texas 77840

Veterinary science has been taught at Texas A & M since 1888. A school of veterinary medicine was established in 1916, the entrance requirement to which was graduation from high school with no less than 15 credits, and graduation from the School of Veteri-Medicine required four years of college study. In 1936, a minimum of 35 semester credits of pre-professional college work was required for enrollment. This was increased to 60 semester credits in 1949, increased to 70 in 1957, decreased to 68 in 1964, and decreased to 66 in 1975.

The professional curriculum was changed from eight required semesters to nine required trimesters in 1964; the curricula now contains 66 pre-professional and 176 professional semester credits.

The school became the College of Veterinary Medicine in August of 1963 when the name of the parent intstitution was changed to Texas A & M University.

First consideration for admission is given to qualified applicants who are residents of Texas. The first year class quota has been filled from this group for many years. If the quota is not filled from that group, a second group of qualified applicants from other states which have no college of veterinary medicine and from foreign countries will be considered on the same basis as the first group. If the quota is not filled from the first two groups, a third group of qualified applicants from other states which have colleges of veterinary medicine will be considered.

There is no separate curriculum in pre-veterinary medicine at Texas A & M University. Students preparing for admission to the professional curriculum in veterinary medicine must choose a specific course of study offered by one of the colleges of the University.

Each student is encouraged to enroll in that degree program that would be their first choice if they do not enter the professional curriculum in veterinary medicine.

The applicant must have an overall grade point ratio of 2.50 or better or a 2.75 grade point ratio or better over the last 45 semester credits completed (A=4.0 grade points).

Each applicant must submit with the application scores attained in the Graduate Record Examination.

A three-member interview team will conduct the applicant interviews. The interview is a structured procedure which seeks to reveal personal characteristics, ability to communicate (proper use of English, organization of thoughts, logic of answers, alertness), motivation for veterinary medicine, maturity, industriousness, diligence, persistence, personality, experiences with animals, seriousness of purpose, knowledge of animals, knowledge of the field of veterinary medicine, and a basis and depth of interest in veterinary medicine as a career.

Three evaluation forms will be given to the applicants who receive an interview. They are to be distributed to the persons best qualified to evaluate the applicant. The Selection Committee will review the completed evaluation forms. The evaluation will include personal traits (motivation, character, industry etc.), recommendation for veterinary school and comments regarding the applicant's special strengths and weaknesses, ability to do independent work, and so forth.

The Selection Committee will review the applicant's application, recommendations and interview, considering the following factors: leadership qualities, extracurricular activites (church, school, community), and employment while a student.

TUFTS UNIVERSITY
School of Veterinary Medicine
Boston, Massachusetts 02111

Tufts opened its doors for its first class of forty-one students in the fall of 1979. The School is dedicated to fulfilling a long-standing need for training veterinarians for the New England states. Contracts for student seats have been negotiated with Connecticut, Maine, Massachusetts, and Rhode Island. Also, a contractual agreement is in effect with New Mexico.

Admissions are based on academic performance in undergraduate college, personal characteristics, scores on Graduate Record Examinations and other relevant factors.

Tufts seeks to enroll students from diverse backgrounds who will actively contribute to the educational community at Tufts, and, of course, to the veterinary profession. A strong background in the sciences, as demonstrated by performance in such areas as biology, chemistry, and physics, is a prerequisite for successful completion of the curriculum. The school is concerned with accepting students whose horizons are broad, and who have demonstrated personal and scholastic achievement.

The Veterinary School has two campuses. One is in the Tufts-New England Medical area of Boston, and the second is in Grafton, Massachusetts. Students will spend their first two years at Tufts-New England studying basic medical sciences with their counterparts from the dental and medical schools. The last two years of clinical training take place at the Grafton campus. Fourth year students will undertake more specialized work in the area of their interest.

Further information can be obtained by writing the School of Veterinary Medicine.

TUSKEGEE INSTITUTE
School of Veterinary Medicine
Tuskegee Institute, Alabama   36088

Authorized by the Board of Trustees of the Institute in 1943, the School of Veterinary Medicine was established at Tuskegee and formal teaching leading to a degree was begun in 1945.

At first, the entrance requirements consisted of a minimum of one year of pre-professional work completed in a recognized college or university with a "C" average or better; effective with the academic year 1949-1950, they were increased to a minimum of two years of pre-professional training.

From the beginning, the professional curriculum has covered four years. The first class was graduated in 1949. The School is considered as a regional service institution for training in veterinary medicine in the South. A maximum of fifty students is admitted each year.

Admission preference is given to applicants from the State of Alabama and to applicants from those cooperating states under the Regional Plan (Arkansas, Georgia, Kentucky, Maryland, Mississippi, North Carolina, South Carolina, Tennessee, Virginia and West Virginia) and other contractual agreements (Guyana and Puerto Rico) for veterinary medical training at Tuskegee Institute. Each of the cooperating states has contracted for a quota of entering first-year students. For the remaining spaces, some preference is given to applicants from states which do not have a veterinary college.

The Committee on Admission in its selection process seeks students who exhibit intellectual, personal, moral, and social traits which are considered most desirable for a doctor of veterinary medicine.

The curriculum and requirements for admission conform to the standards set forth by the American Veterinary Medical Association. To be considered for admission to the School of Veterinary Medicine, applicants must present a total of not less than two pre-professional years of college credit (60 semester credits or 90 quarter credits) which have been completed with at least a "C" average or its equivalent in a recognized college or university.

Persons who do not include Animal and Poultry Science courses in their pre-professional studies may be admitted at the discretion of the Admission Committee to the School of Veterinary Medicine, if they have fulfilled all other requirements. Such individuals must, in every case, complete these courses prior to attaining third-year status in the School of Veterinary Medicine. This exception does not mean that an applicant may present less than 60 semester or 90 quarter credits for admission. Where Animal and Poultry Science courses have not been included in the pre-professional studies, the applicant must have completed a corresponding number of additional credits in the elective categories. Courses required in the professional veterinary curriculum cannot be used to satisfy elective admission requirements.

Application for admission may be secured by writing to the Admissions Office of the Institute or the Dean of the School of Veterinary Medicine.

Out-of-state applicants are advised to contact the officials listed below for their respective states.

Arkansas
    Dean, College of Agriculture and
        Home Economics
    University of Arkansas
    Fayetteville, Arkansas   72701

Georgia
    Associate Executive Secretary
    Regents of the University System of Georgia
    244 Washington St., SW
    Atlanta, Georgia   30330

Kentucky
    Chairman
    Kentucky Regional Education Certification
        Committee
    University of Kentucky
    Lexington, Kentucky 40506

Maryland
    Director of Admissions
    University of Maryland
    College Park, Maryland 20740

Mississippi
    Executive Secretary
    Board of Trustees of Higher Learning
    1855 Eastover Drive
    PO Box 2336
    Jackson, Mississippi 39211

North Carolina
    Secretary
    North Carolina Veterinary Certification
        Committee
    School of Agriculture and Life Sciences
    North Carolina State University
    Raleigh, North Carolina 27607

South Carolina
    Secretary
    Regional Education Board
    Rm 208 Rutledge Building
    Columbia, South Carolina 29201

Tennessee
    Chairman, Certification Committee
    Regional Program for Veterinary Training
    College of Agriculture
    University of Tennessee
    Knoxville, Tennessee 38916

Virginia
> State Certification Officer
> Virginia Council of Higher Education
> 700 Fidelity Building
> 9th and Main Streets
> Richmond, Virginia 23219

West Virginia
> Dean, College of Agriculture
> Forestry and Home Economics
> West Virginia University
> Morgantown, West Virginia 26506

VIRGINIA POLYTECHNIC INSTITUTE AND STATE UNIVERSITY
College of Veterinary Medicine
Blacksburg, Virginia 24061

The Veterinary College at Virginia Tech will admit its first class in the fall of 1980. Preference in admission will be given to Virginia residents and to residents of states with which contractual arrangements have been made.

The student entering the veterinary medical college must show evidence of intellectual ability and achievement as well as suitable personal qualities. Because the number of applicants greatly exceeds the number of places in the entering class, only those who demonstrate these qualifications to a high degree will be selected.

Applications will be accepted from those who have completed a minimum of 90 quarter credit hours, including all required courses. These requirements must be met by the end of the spring term of the year for which application is being made. Exceptional students with the minimum college course work are encouraged to apply.

Applicants achieving a grade point average of 2.8 or above (A=4.0) on all college credit work will be given first consideration by the Admissions Committee.

For further information, write to:

Virginia Polytechnic Institute and State
  University
College of Veterinary Medicine
Blacksburg, Virginia 24061.

WASHINGTON STATE UNIVERSITY
College of Veterinary Medicine
Pullman, Washington 99163

In 1890, the legislature of the State of Washington authorized the establishment of the State Agricultural College, Experiment Station and School of Science, now officially designated as Washington State University. One of the major subjects to be taught was veterinary art.

In 1899 the School of Veterinary Science was made a major division of the College, and courses leading to the professional degree were offered. Two years of high school credit were required for admission, and three years of professional study qualified one for the degree, Doctor of Veterinary Medicine. The administrative officer was known as head of the department.

In 1906 high school graduation was required for admission, and four years of study were required for graduation. Reorganization of the State College occurred in 1917, and the deaprtment was then administered by a dean. In 1925 the name of the division was changed to College of Veterinary Medicine.

In 1935 one year of specified college credit was required for admission; in 1949 this was increased to two years. Pre-veterinary requirements are currently a minimum of three years.

A regional program initiated with Idaho (1974) and with Oregon (1977) is referred to as the Washington-Oregon-Idaho Regional Program in Veterinary Medicine (WOI). In general, first admissions preference is given to qualified students who are residents of these states.

Second preference is given to qualified students certified by compact states, and third preference to all other qualified students. The third preference group is utilized only under the very rarest of circumstances.

The College of Veterinary Medicine at Washington State University has entered into a regional education program with the states of Alaska, Arizona, Hawaii, Montana, Nevada, New Mexico, Utah, and Wyoming. Under the terms of the compact, a certified student admitted from one of these states is sponsored financially by his home state and is subject only to fees for resident Washington students. Students must apply to their home states for certification, in addition to making application to the Director of Admissions at Washington State University. Additional information regarding regional veterinary education may be obtained from the following:

> The Executive Director
> Western Interstate Commission for Higher Education
> PO Drawer P
> Boulder, Colorado 80302.

Applicants for admission to the College of Veterinary Medicine should present at least 90 semester hours of acceptable credits from a recognized college or university. The 90 semester hours must include courses that will meet the general university requirements for graduation.

Each applicant must supply satisfactory evidence of completion of all pre-veterinary requirements by the end of the current academic year. A minimum overall grade point average of 3.00 (on a 4.00 system) covering academic work equivalent to that taught at Washington State University will normally be required for consideration for admission. Exceptions to this rule may be students who have compiled a minimum basic science (biological and physical science) GPA of 3.00 or have shown outstanding improvement over the last two years of academic work, i.e. performance at the 3.50 level over this period. However, graduate performance will be evaluated carefully, both in terms of workload and total course load, since graduate course grades generally fall only in the A-B category. In all cases, a student should provide sufficient evidence that he or she can handle a full course load. This means an average of at least 15 credit hours per term. Preference will be given candidates with the greater depth and breadth of academic background.

The average student selected for admission will have completed four years of pre-veterinary medical education. However, qualified juniors are encouraged to apply. Scores from the General Aptitude and Advanced Test Biology section of the Graduate Record Examination will be included in the assessment of the applicant's scholastic achievement.

In order to gain serious consideration an applicant should have been employed by, worked on a volunteer basis for, or by some other means gained significant contact with a graduate veterinarian. Significant contact will be established by the terms of a favorable letter of evaluation from said veterinarian or veterinarians. Applicants should endeavor to record a minimum of 300 hours of such experience. Veterinary contact in connection with normal farming or ranching operations or in treatment of applicant's pets will be considered beneficial but, by itself, insufficient to meet the terms of this particular criterion. Additional animal experience will improve an applicant's credentials.

Each applicant should have three recommendation forms submitted to the Admissions Committee as an aid in evaluation of personal traits. The opinions of individuals within the veterinary medical profession, or in closely allied areas, are considered of greatest value to the Committee. The individuals selected should know the applicant well so that the recommendations will be meaningful.

Achievements, leadership ability, and participation in constructive activities outside formal academic areas will receive consideration. Determination, motivation, responsibility and maturity are also considered by the Committee.

    Candidates should demonstrate during the interview that they are articulate, poised, and well motivated toward a career in veterinary medicine. Interviews are scheduled and conducted at the discretion of the Admissions Committee and will normally be conducted on the Washington State University Campus.

SUMMARY ON ADMISSIONS

It should be noted here that with the many schools throughout the country, the really determined student should be able to surmount his particular difficulties and get an education in veterinary medicine.

It is true, of course, that degrees can be obtained in foreign schools. These may cause the individuals some problems, particularly of they intend to practice in the United States. But this course to a DVM degree has been taken successfully, and offers many unique opportunities. Some of the foreign schools provide excellent educations, but the student must naturally have a fluency in the language of the country.

There is a great tendency these days to encourage new professional graduates in any profession to go into a specialty, or an advanced post-doctoral degree. I have mixed emotions on this. I tend to believe some specialties do require advanced post-doctoral education, while others do not. An individual can, of course, fall into the trap of becoming a "professional student."

A post-doctoral education can be obtained in any one of the academic areas listed previously. For example, the new Doctor of Veterinary Medicine may decide to specialize in microbiology or public health and take a Masters or a Ph.D. degree in either one.

It is doubtful if you would need that additional education for most positions or practices calling for a veterinarian. Remember, just because you get more degrees than a thermometer doesn't mean you're hot! However, most universities that have veterinary schools will have a selection of post-doctoral programs and the student will have plenty of time to choose.

Do what <u>you</u> want to do. Don't let advisors and peers talk you into doing what they want!

VETERINARY SCIENCE PROGRAMS

Following is a listing of veterinary programs in the United States. These programs include those leading to Bachelor's, Master's and Ph.D. degrees in allied veterinary fields such as parasitology, animal pathology, etc. The degrees granted by these institutions are not DVM degrees, but are in areas that lend support to the veterinary doctor, particularly in the field of research.

Arizona
    Department of Veterinary Science
    University of Arizona
    Tucson, Arizona 85721

Arkansas
    Department of Animal Sciences
    University of Arkansas
    Fayetteville, Arkansas 72701

Colorado
    College of Veterinary Medicine
    and Biomedical Sciences
    Colorado State University
    Fort Collins, Colorado 80523

Connecticut
    Department of Pathobiology
    University of Connecticut
    Storrs, Connecticut 06268

Delaware
    Department of Animal Science
    and Agricultural Biochemistry
    College of Agricultural Sciences
    University of Delaware
    Newark, Delaware 19711

Idaho
>Department of Veterinary Science
>University of Idaho
>Moscow, Idaho 83843

Kentucky
>Department of Veterinary Science
>University of Kentucky
>Lexington, Kentucky 40506

Maine
>Department of Animal and Veterinary Sciences
>134 Hitchner Hall
>University of Maine
>Orono, Maine 04473

Maryland
>Department of Veterinary Science
>University of Maryland
>College Park, Maryland 20740

Massachusetts
>Department of Veterinary and Animal Science
>University of Massachusetts
>Amherst, Massachusetts 01002

Montana
>Veterinary Research Laboratory and Department of Veterinary Science
>Montana State University
>Bozeman, Montana 59715

Nebraska
>Department of Veterinary Science
>University of Nebraska
>Lincoln, Nebraska 68583

Nevada
: Division of Veterinary Medicine
University of Nevada
5305 Mill Street
Reno, Nevada 89507

New Hampshire
: Department of Animal Sciences
University of New Hampshire, Kendall Hall
Durham, New Hampshire 03824

New Jersey
: Cook College
Rutgers University
The State University of New Jersey
New Brunswick, New Jersey 08903

North Carolina
: Department of Veterinary Science
North Carolina State University
Raleigh, North Carolina 27607

North Dakota
: Veterinary Science Department
North Dakota State University of Agriculture
  and Applied Sciences
Fargo, North Dakota 58102

Ohio
: Department of Veterinary Science
Ohio Agricultural Research and Development
  Center
Wooster, Ohio 44691

Oregon
: Department of Veterinary Medicine
Oregon State University
Corvallis, Oregon 97331

Pennsylvania
    Department of Veterinary Science
    The Pennsylvania State University
    University Park, Pennsylvania 16802

Puerto Rico
    Department of Animal Industry
    College of Agricultural Sciences
    Mayaquez Campus
    Mayaquez, Puerto Rico 00708

Rhode Island
    Department of Animal Pathology
    University of Rhode Island
    Kingston, Rhode Island 02881

South Dakota
    Department of Veterinary Science
    Animal Disease Research and Diagnostic
      Laboratory
    South Dakota State University
    Brookings, South Dakota 57007

Utah
    Department of Animal, Dairy, and Veterinary
      Science
    Utah State University
    Logan, Utah 84322

Vermont
    Department of Animal Pathology
    University of Vermont
    Burlington, Vermont 05401

Virginia
    Department of Veterinary Science
    Virginia Polytechnic Institute and State
      University
    Blacksburg, Virginia 24061

West Virginia
> Division of Animal and Veterinary Science
> Agriculture Science Building, Rm G036
> Evansdale Campus
> West Virginia University
> Morgantown, West Virginia 26505

Wisconsin
> Department of Veterinary Science
> University of Wisconsin
> 1655 Linden Drive
> Madison, Wisconsin 53706

Wyoming
> Division of Microbiology and Veterinary
>   Medicine
> PO Box 3354, University Station
> Laramie, Wyoming 82071

It is also suggested that the interested student contact the colleges of veterinary medicine for information on pre-professional veterinary programs that lead to a Bachelor's degree.

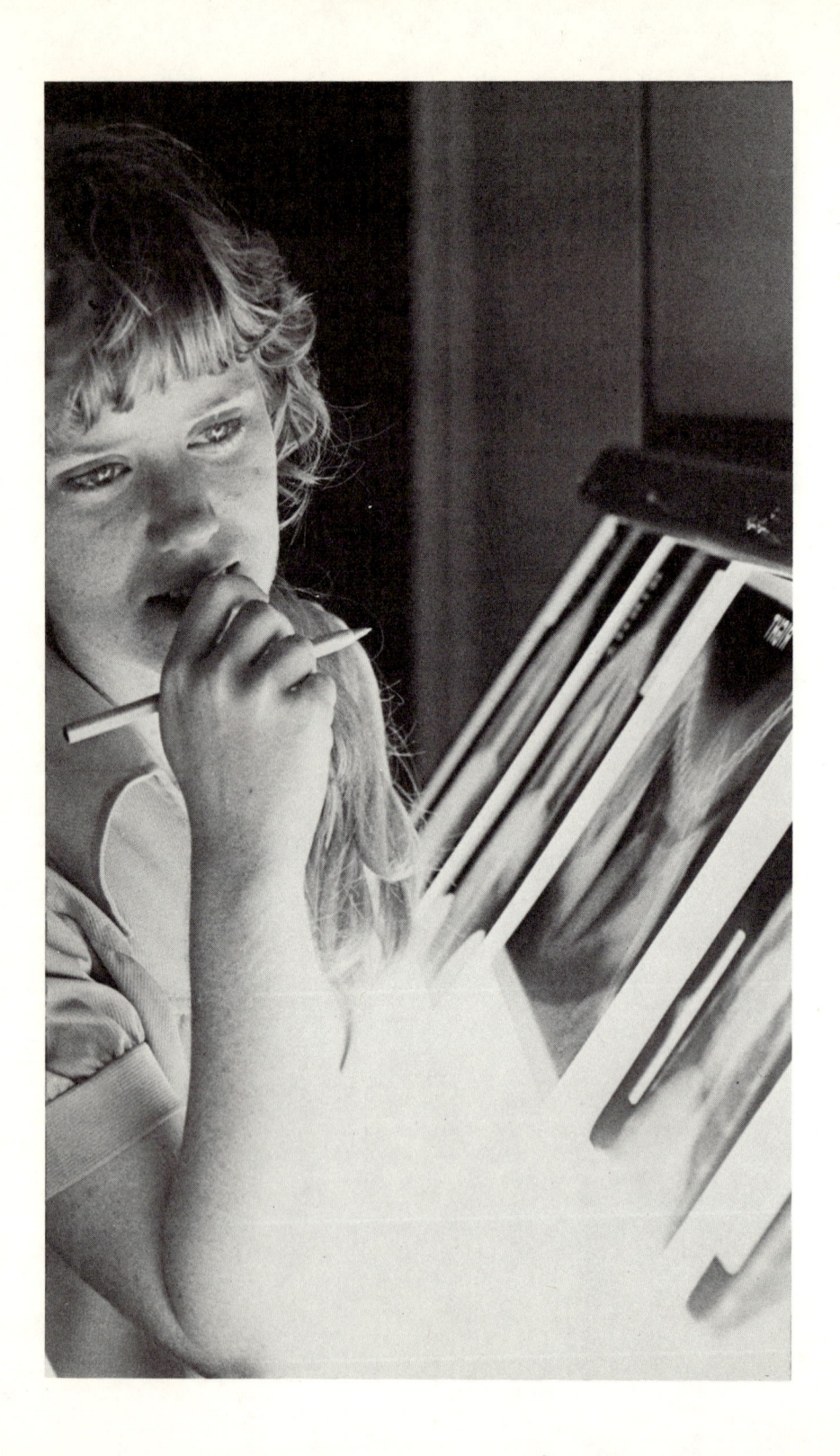

CHAPTER 5
Introduction to Allied Animal Health Careers

Many young men and women simply do not wish to pursue the degree of Doctor of Veterinary Medicine. And today they can find satisfying and rewarding careers in auxiliary fields such as veterinary health technology, animal welfare, laboratory animal technology and wildlife conservation.

The American Veterinary Medical Association has recognized the increasing need for personnel qualified by formal training to assist in veterinary practices, biological laboratories, animal research, food inspection, and other areas where science and animals are combined.

As the animal health care system becomes more complex, more technical assistance will be needed to free practicing veterinarians to spend more time with clients and patients.

Professionals representing public health organizations, research institutions, pharmaceutical manufacturers, and universities express a need for technicians with specialized training concerned with animal health and animal care. Non-professional people have been, and are now employed in this type of work after various kinds of on-the-job training.

The intent of the formal academic programs is to supply a pool of potential employees with a background designed to minimize the time and effort necessary to adapt them to particular job situations.

A number of colleges have recently developed two and four year programs which provide students with the knowledge and skills needed to assist veterinarians in clinical practice, laboratory animal care, zoo medicine, diagnostic work and research. And graduates of these programs are valuable and critically necessary parts of the animal health care field. Just imagine a human hospital without nurses or laboratory specialists!

ANIMAL HEALTH TECHNOLOGIST

The division between the animal health techno*logist* and the animal health tech*nician* is difficult to discern. Many of the duties seem to overlap. The main difference lies in the opportunities for advancement. Supervisory positions are more available to the tech*nologist* than to the tech*nician*.

Animal health technology is a four year college program leading to a Bachelor of Science degree. The individual is trained in the routines of animal care, plus nutrition, breeding, and in the treatment and prevention of animal diseases. Diagnostic procedures and surgical assistance are studied. The technologist can perform any type of clinical work with animals as long as there is supervision by a veterinarian. A technologist might administer anesthesia or take X-rays or do blood work. He cannot, however, make diagnoses, or perform surgery, or prescribe medicine independently of a veterinarian, but he does assist the veterinarian in all of these functions.

A technologist, can, with the Bachelor of Science degree, work in an animal hospital, a research laboratory, a zoo, museum, or wildlife perserve. Food and drug companies also employ animal health technologists, and in organizations such as these, the graduate of the four-year program is prepared to hold supervisory positions.

There are only a limited number of four-year programs simply because the demand for the graduates is small. Whereas the need for animal "nurses" (technicians) is large, the need for "supervisors" (technologists) - or those whose education would indicate management ability and desire - is more restricted. In most cases, where the technician's duties leave off, those of the professionally trained veterinarian take over, and there is only a limited area for personnel between the two.

Not unlike the prospective veterinarian, the prospective animal technologist should possess a high degree of tenacity. Jobs at the zoo, in wildlife conservation, and the like do exist, but their numbers are restricted, and although highly rewarding, they can be difficult to locate.

ANIMAL HEALTH TECHNICIAN

An animal health technician is the veterinarian's assistant, and functions in much the same way as does a nurse in human medicine. The technician is trained in a two-year college program that gives an associate degree in applied science. Most programs admit holders of high school diplomas or equivalency certificates on an individual basis. Items considered in selection of applicants include aptitude, interest, and ability of the applicant to profit from the courses offered. Specific entrance requirements may be determined by inquiry directed to the school which the student plans to attend. Generally, a strong background in high school science courses is advantageous.

The degree requires completion of general courses in biology, chemistry, communications, mathematics, economics, and business management, as well as specific courses covering such subjects as physiology, nutrition, microbiology, parsitology, animal care, laboratory procedures, clinical techniques, radiology, toxicology, ethics, and client relations. The specific courses are usually taught by experienced veterinarians who are aware of what the technician's future employers will expect him or her to know.

The following is a typical curriculum outline.

1st Semester	Hours
Orientation	2

Mathematics	3
Anatomy and Physiology	5
Microbiology	4
Terminology	2
total	16

2nd Semester

Laboratory Procedures I	3
Chemistry	4
Office Procedures	3
Sanitation and Hygiene	3
Nutrition	3
total	16

3rd Semester

Clinical Procedures I	3
English	3
Laboratory Procedures II	4
Clinical Pathology	4
Special Project	2
total	16

4th Semester

Clinical Procedures II	4
Speech	2
Research Techniques	3
Laboratory Animal Science	4
Reproduction	3
total	16

Practical experience with live animals and field experience under actual working conditions are intergral parts of most technician programs. Many programs allow for some elective courses to meet special interests of certain students and some use the summer period between semester for part of the instructional program.

All programs for training animal health technicians are designed to provide background knowledge and basic skills upon which to build when the graduates, at their various places of employment, begin to learn the specific procedures which they will be called upon to perform. Most programs lead to an Associate of Arts or an Associate in Applied Sciences degree.

The deliniation between the technologist and technician is defined to such a limited extent that the two titles - "technologist" and "technician" - are often used interchangeably. However, the associate-degreed technician will frequently be limited by his training and education to the role of the assistant.

The registration provisions of animal health technicians vary from state to state, according to the individual governments' needs and laws. For the most part, the licensing practices of the states do not differentiate between the animal technologist and the technician.

TECHNOLOGY PROGRAM SUMMARY

An animal health technician is described an a person knowledgeable in the care and handling of animals, in the basic principles of normal and abnormal life processes, and in routine laboratory and clinical procedures. He is primarily an assistant to veterinarians, biological research workers, and other scientists.

Examples of duties which are performed by animal health technicians as assistants to practicing veterinarians include:
- obtaining and recording information about cases
- preparation of patients, instruments, equipment, and medicaments for surgery
- collection of speciments and performance of certain laboratory procedures
- application of wound dressings

- assisting a veterinarian in diagnostic, medical, and surgical procedures

In general, the duties of an animal health technician in a veterinary practice may include any part of the practice which does not involve diagnostic, prescriptive, or surgical procedures, and whose performance by a technician is not in conflict with the state practice act. All functions of an animal health technician are performed under the supervision of a veterinarian. The veterinarian or the veterinary practice which employs an animal health technician is responsible for the acts of the technician and for his compensation.

Animal health technicians are employed in a number of other situations in addition to veterinary practices. Laboratories doing biological research, companies producing drugs or feeds, animal production facilities, zoos, and meat packing companies are examples of organizations that may have need for the special skills of animal health technicians. Duties performed in such places may include:
- record keeping
- animal care and feeding
- performance of laboratory procedures
- maintenance of equipment and products
- inspection of products or carcasses.

In such employment the animal health technician works under the supervision of a scientist or a senior technologist. In no case is animal health technology practiced as an independent venture.

The animal health technician or technologist can expect a salary range from approximately $8,000 per annum to $18,000.

In addition to the programs discussed, colleges of agriculture and many other institutions offer degree programs in animal husbandry, various biological sciences, and other animal-related fields which must provide the basic supporting matrix of which the veterinarian is only a part.

ACCREDITATION OF TECHNOLOGY PROGRAMS

Because the veterinary-related careers are so new, there are still some problems associated with them. For example, training varies widely from school to school. Not all programs meet the same standards or have the same objectives. There are very few standard textbooks or uniform exams for animal health technician subjects. The schools and programs vary so much that a veterinarian wishing to hire an animal health technician does not really know how well an applicant has been trained or what his or her capabilities are. The licensing laws that apply to animal health technicians also need to be clarified and defined.

To solve these problems, the American Veterinary Medical Association has established basic standards that must be met by a school in order for the school's animal health technician program to be accredited (that is, "approved"). If an individual completes an accredited program, it means that the school has taught him or her basic subjects according to certain standards.

To be accredited by the American Veterinary Medical Association, a program in animal health technology must meet the following minimum requirements:
- it must be a part of an accredited institution of higher learning
- it must be on a sound financial basis
- it must conduct itself in an ethical manner
- the physical plant and equipment must be adequate for the purposes intended
- the number of students enrolled must be in keeping with the size of the facility and the faculty
- library facilities must be adequate
- admission requirements for students must include high school graduation or equivalent,

good character, initiative, and motivation
- the faculty must be fully qualified in the subject areas to be taught
- the curriculum must provide a sound foundation in basic animal technology, and develop habits of mind that will inspire the student to continue to educate himself and to be educated
- it must cover at least two academic years and must include basic general college level courses, as well as specific job-oriented courses to be taught in laboratory and clinical settings with the use of live animals; specific courses must be taught on a very practical plane with the intent of making the student a useful assistant
- a system must be established to evaluate the activities of the graduates of the programs
- effort must be made to provide opportunities for continuing education for employed animal technicians.

The following list includes the names and addresses of some institutions that currently offer an animal health technician training program that has been accredited by the American Veterinary Medical Association, or which they believe may be potentially accreditable.

The AVMA has evaluated a number of animal health technology programs and accredited those which meet standards they believe essential for adequate training in this field . The accrediting procedure is designed to assure both interested students and prospective employers that certain schools offer what the AVMA considers to be proper training in animal health technology. Graduation from an accredited training program is also required for registration in an increasing number of states.

Programs currently accredited are indicated on the list. The AVMA's accreditation procedure is still relatively new, and they believe there probably are several good programs that have not yet been evaluated. Therefore, non-accredited programs on this list should not necessarily be considered inferior. However, the AVMA does not in any way approve or endorse any animal health technology program other than those designated on this list as "accredited."

An individual is encouraged to enter a program that has been accredited by the AVMA. If this is not possible, it is urged that her or she enroll in a two-year program at an accredited institution of higher learning where instruction is given in laboratory and clinical settings, and live animals are available for instruction.

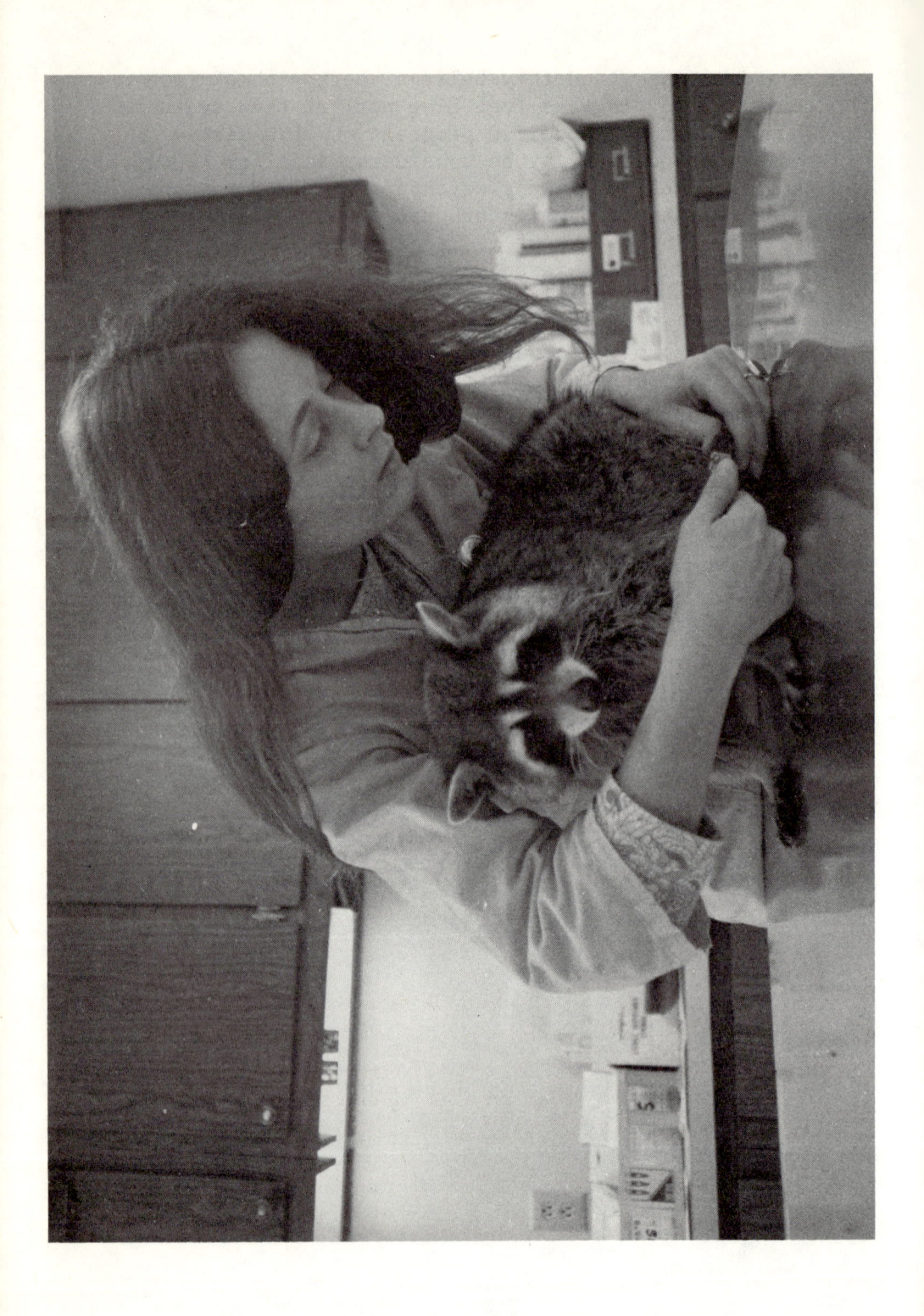

CHAPTER 6
Animal Health Technology Programs

It should be noted that the schools designated by the asterisk (*) were accredited by the time of publication. Since that time, more may have received accreditation from the AVMA. The AVMA may be contacted for an up-to-date listing. Please write:

The American Veterinary Medical Association
930 North Meacham Road
Schaumburg, Illinois 60196.

Unless otherwise indicated, the following schools are two-year programs.

Alabama
    Snead State Junior College
    Animal Hospital Technology Program
    Boaz, Alabama 35957

California
    Hartnell College
    Animal Health Technician Program
    156 Homestead Avenue
    Salinas, California 93901

    Los Angeles Pierce College *
    Animal Health Technology Program
    6201 Winnetka Avenue
    Woodland Hills, California 92101

    Yuba College
    Animal Health Technician Program
    Yuba Community College
    Maryville, California 95901

Mt. San Antonio College *
Animal Health Technology Program
1100 North Grand Avenue
Walnut, California 91789

San Diego Mesa College
Animal Health Technology Program
7250 Mesa College Drive
San Diego, California 92111

Colorado
    Colorado Mountain College *
    Animal Health Technology Program
    West Campus
    Glenwood Springs, Colorado 81601

    Bel-Rea Institute of Animal Technology *
    9870 East Alameda
    Denver, Colorado 80231

Connecticut
    Quinnipiac College
    Hamden, Connecticut 06518
    (4 year program)

Florida
    St. Petersburg Junior College
    Animal Science Technology Program
    Box 13489
    St. Petersburg, Florida 33733

Georgia
    Abraham Baldwin Agriculture College *
    Animal Health Technology Program
    Tifton, Georgia 31794

    Fort Valley State College
    Animal Health Technology Program
    Fort Valley, Georgia 31030

Illinois
    Parkland College *
    Veterinary Technology Program
    2400 Bradley
    Champaign, Illinois   61820

Indiana
    School of Veterinary Medicine *
    Veterinary Technology Program
    Purdue University
    West Lafayette, Indiana   47907

Kansas
    Colby Community College *
    Animal Technology Program
    1255 South Range
    Colby, Kansas   67701

Kentucky
    Morehead State University
    Veterinary Technology Program
    Box 702
    Morehead, Kentucky   40351

Louisiana
    Department of Agricultural Sciences
    Veterinary Technology Program
    Northwestern State University of Louisiana
    Natchitoches, Louisiana   71457

Maine
    Department of Animal and Veterinary Sciences
    Animal Medical Technology Program
    University of Maine
    Orono, Maine   04473

Maryland
>	Essex Community College
>	Animal Science Technician Program
>	7201 Rossville Boulevard
>	Baltimore, Maryland 21237
>
>	Garrett Community College
>	Veterinary Science Technology Program
>	PO Box 151
>	McHenry, Maryland 21541

Massachusetts
>	Department of Veterinary and Animal Sciences
>	Laboratory Animal Technology Program
>	Stockbridge School of Agriculture
>	University of Massachusetts
>	Amherst, Massachusetts 01001
>
>	Department of Veterinary and Animal Sciences
>	Veterinary and Animal Science Career Program
>	Holyoke Community College
>	303 Homestead Avenue
>	Holyoke, Massachusetts 01040
>
>	Becker Junior College
>	Veterinary Assistant Program
>	1003 Old Main Street
>	Leicester, Massachusetts 01524
>
>	Holliston Junior College *
>	Rogers Road
>	Holliston, Massachusetts 01746

Michigan
>	Wayne State University *
>	School of Medicine
>	Animal Health Technology Program
>	540 Canfield
>	Detroit, Michigan 48201

College of Veterinary Medicine *
Animal Technology Program
Michigan State University
East Lansing, Michigan 48823

Minnesota
Medical Institute of Minnesota
2309 Nicollet Avenue
Minneapolis, Minnesota 55404

University of Minnesota *
Animal Health Technology Program
Waseca, Minnesota 56093

Mississippi
Hinds Junior College
Animal Technician Program
Raymond, Mississippi 39154

Missouri
Maple Woods Community College *
Animal Health Technology Program
2601 N E Barry Road
Kansas City, Missouri 64156

Jefferson College
Animal Health Technology Program
Hillsboro, Missouri 63050

Animal Health Technology Program
Northeast Missouri State University
Kirksville, Missouri 63501

Nebraska
School of Technical Agriculture *
University of Nebraska
Veterinary Technology Program
Curtis, Nebraska 69025

New Jersey
>	Camden County College
>	Animal Science Technology Program
>	PO Box 200
>	Blackwood, New Jersey 08010

New York
>	Veterinary Science Technology Department
>	Canton Agricultural & Technical College
>	Canton, New York 13617
>
>	Department of Biological Sciences
>	State University of New York
>	Agriculture and Technical College
>	Farmingdale, New York 11735
>
>	Veterinary Science Technology Department *
>	Agricultural and Technical College
>	State University of New York
>	Delhi, New York 13753

North Carolina
>	Central Carolina Technical Institute *
>	Veterinary Medical Technology Program
>	Route 2, Box 55
>	Sanford, North Carolina 27330

North Dakota
>	North Dakota State University
>	Animal Health Technician Program
>	Department of Veterinary Science
>	Fargo, North Dakota 58102

Ohio
>	Columbus Technical Institute *
>	Animal Health Technology Program
>	550 East Springs Street
>	Columbus, Ohio 43215

Raymond Walters College *
Animal Health Technology Program
University of Cincinnati
Cincinnati, Ohio 45221

Oklahoma
    Murray State College
    Veterinary Assistant Technology Program
    Tishomingo, Oklahoma 73460

Oregon
    Portland Community College
    Veterinary Science Technology Program
    Portland, Oregon 97208

Pennsylvania
    Harcum Junior College *
    Animal Technician Program
    Bryn Mawr, Pennsylvania 19010

    Median School
    Animal Health Technology Program
    12 - 8th Street
    Pittsburgh, Pennsylvania 15222

South Carolina
    Tri-County Technical College
    Veterinary Assistant Technology Program
    PO Box 587
    Pendleton, South Carolina 29670

Tennessee
    Columbia State Community College
    Animal Hospital Technology Program
    Columbia, Tennessee 38491

Texas
- Mountain View College
Animal Medical Technology Program
4849 W. Illinois Avenue
Dallas, Texas 75211

- Texas State Technical College *
Animal Medical Technology Program
James Connally Campus
Waco, Texas 76705

- Frank Phillips College
Animal Health Technology Program
Box 111
Borger, Texas 79007

- Range Animal Science Department
Animal Technology Program
Sul Ross State University
Alpine, Texas 78839

- Biomedical Science Program
Department of Veterinary Public Health
College of Veterinary Medicine
Texas A & M University
College Station, Texas 77943
(4 year program)

Virginia
- Blue Ridge Community College *
Animal Technology Program
Box 80
Weyers Cave, Virginia 24486

- Northern Virginia Community College
Animal Science Technology Program
Loudoun Campus
1000 Harry Flood Bryd Highway
Sterling, Virginia 22170

Washington
    Fort Steilacoom Community College *
    Animal Technology Program
    6010 Mount Tacoma Drive, S.W.
    Tacoma, Washington 98499

West Virginia
    Fairmont State College
    Veterinary Assistant Program
    Fairmont, West Virginia 26554

Wisconsin
    Madison Area Technical College *
    Animal Technician Program
    211 North Carroll Street
    Madison, Wisconsin 53703

Wyoming
    Eastern Wyoming College *
    Animal Health Technology Program
    3200 West C. Street
    Torrington, Wyoming 82240

    Wyoming School of Animal Technology
    PO Box 872
    Thermopolis, Wyoming 82443

CHAPTER 7
Laboratory Health Technician

There is a large career field in the area of laboratory animal science. Although very few of the colleges named in the listing of animal health technology programs (preceeding chapter) specialize in laboratory animal care, some do.

Laboratory animal technicians and technologists are employed by medical, dental and veterinary schools, hospitals, the pharmaceuticals industry, food production companies, research institutes, breeders of laboratory animals, government agencies, diagnostic and testing laboratories, and public health agencies.

The technician or technologist generally works in one of the following areas: animal husbandry (including the daily care, breeding, and feeding of the different kinds of animals used in laboratories), laboratory animal technology or as an animal health technician.

Laboratory animal technology includes procedures performed with animals in laboratory work. Some of these tasks are giving injections, taking samples of various body fluids or tissues, observing reactions of animals to different tests, making chemical analyses, taking physiological recordings and providing animal care.

The laboratory animal technician or technologist works under the direction of professional personnel such as veterinarians, physiologists, or microbiologists, and is usually able to work with a wider range of animals than does the animal health technician employed by a veterinary practice. Species used in research include mice, rats, guinea pigs, rabbits, dogs, cats, non-human primates, fish, birds, and some farm animals. Most facilities engaged in research offer on-the-job training geared toward national certification.

While animal health technicians are usually state-registered, the American Association for Laboratory Science (AALAS) certified individuals are not. At the technologist level there is a national registry published by and available from the national office.

The Animal Technician Certification Board (ATCB) of the American Association for Laboratory Animal Science provides examinations and national certification for laboratory animal personnel who are eligible and employed in laboratory animal facilities. The examinations administered by the ATCB are offered at three levels: 1) Assistant Laboratory Animal Technician (one year of experience required); 2) Laboratory Animal Technician (three years of experience required); and 3) Laboratory Animal Technologist (six years of experience required).

Applications for certification are available from

The American Association for Laboratory Animal
  Science
2317 W. Jefferson St. Suite 208
Joliet, Illinois 60435.

ANIMAL TECHNICIAN CERTIFICATION BOARD EXAMINATIONS

An assistant laboratory animal technician would be examined on this material:
- basic structure and function of body systems
- nutrition
- genetics and mating systems
- animal handling, restraint, and identification
- equipment and materials: identification, maintenance and proper use
- sanitation and hygiene
- animal health and disease
- animal nursing
- animal experimental techniques.

Upon certification, the individual is recognized as

being capable of the following minimum skills. He must be:
- aware of federal, state and local regulations pertaining to laboratory animals and know where to obtain additional or current regulatory information
- able to observe or detect alterations in animal room enviorment, including temperature, air exchange and light cycles
- able to recognize common signs of clinical illness in laboratory animals
- able to provide care of laboratory animals in a safe and sanitary manner using equipment under established procedures
- able to handle, restrain, and determine the sex of all common laboratory animals
- capable of assisting with various methods of animal identification and maintenance of accurate records
- able to observe and report irregularities in laboratory animals, including variations in dietary habits, abnormal stool or urine specimens, unusual behavior and death
- able to provide general technical assistance for a supervisor or investigator
- able to provide routine treatments as instructed, including procedures such as ear mite medication and clipping of overgrown teeth
- knowledgeable concerning personal hygiene and various sanitation procedures.

A laboratory animal technician would be examined on:
- anatomy, physiology, and related disorders
- nutrition and metabolism
- genetics and mating systems
- physiological parameters, breeds, strains, and behavioral traits
- veterinary pharmacology, anesthesia, euthanasia
- animal health and disease

- housing and equipment design
- sanitation, hygiene and safety
- administration, management and record keeping
- shipping and receiving animals
- gnotobiology and germfree animal techniques
- animal experimentation techniques.

Upon certification, the individual is recognized as being capable of minimum skills. In addition to the capabilities of an assistant laboratory technician, the laboratory technician must be:
- capable of providing leadership and direction for assigned assistant laboratory animal technicians
- knowledgeable regarding basic anesthetic principles and procedures for common laboratory animals
- able to perform preoperative procedures and postoperative care as directed
- able to maintain accurate records on animal colonies
- able to maintain accurate supply and equipment inventories for an assigned area
- capable of administering oral, intramuscular, intraperitoneal, subcutaneous or intravenous medication as directed
- able to obtain blood, urine, or fecal samples, and rectal or nasal swabs from common laboratory animals
- capable of supplying technical services to investigators, including mixing and dispensing special diets, medicating drinking water, providing special housing requirements, or assisting with specific restraint and handling procedures.

A laboratory animal technologist would be examined on:
- basic concepts in the sciences
- comparative anatomy, physiology, and related disorders

- administration, management and record keeping
- housing and equipment design
- shipping and receiving animals
- sanitation, hygiene and safety
- nutrition and metabolism
- genetics and mating systems
- physiological parameters, breeds, strains, and behavioral traits
- handling and identification
- animal experimental techniques
- gnotobiology and germfree animal techniques
- radiology
- animal health and disease
- veterinary pharmacology
- veterinary anesthesia and euthanasia
- surgical nursing
- veterinary clinical pathology in the areas of parasitology, hematology, urinalysis, mycology, bacteriology.

Upon certification, the individual is recognized as being capable of minimum skills. In addition to the capabilities of a laboratory animal technician, the laboratory animal technologist must be:
- knowledgeable concerning basic management and administration of animal facilities including:
  - fiscal matters involving budgeting, cost accounting and purchasing
  - giving daily work assignments and instructions
  - responsibility for accurate inventories of animal care equipment and supplies
  - thorough familiarity with the operation and maintenance of animal care equipment
- knowledgeable in facility design, cage requirements and work flow patterns with abilities to assist in facility renovation or building programs and updating or purchasing equipment
- familiar with the reproductive patterns and rearing of common laboratory animals

- knowledgeable concerning basic principles of of primatology, including handling, restraint, reproductive patterns, tuberculin testing schedules and quarantine procedures
- able to administer effective anesthetic drugs or provide approved euthanasia for various laboratory animals
- knowledgeable regarding anatomic and physiologic perculiarities of laboratory animals, with the ability to select appropriate species for specific research studies
- able to provide aseptic support, perform minor surgical procedures, assist with surgery, and supervise or provide preoperative and postoperative care as prescribed
- knowledgeable concerning principles of disease transmission, prevention and control
- capable of maintaining gnotobiotic animals, quarantine wards, prevention and control
- aware of basic nutrient requirements of the various laboratory animal species
- knowledgeable concerning personnel safety, radiation control and biohazard containment
- able to assist in instruction and training of laboratory animals technicians
- informed concerning current animal welfare legislation and trends in the use of humane aspects of laboratory animals
- able to assist in collecting date for preparation of the Annual Animal Welfare Report.